# Around We Go

## By

## Tonya L. Chatelain

ISBN: 1-4033-1376-8 (Electronic)
ISBN: 1-4033-1377-6 (Softcover)

This book is printed on acid free paper.

1stBooks – rev. 5/22/02

*Tiffany had never experienced anything like this before. She was not sure of her feelings or even if those feelings were what she wanted and needed, until she met Susan. Susan was what she wanted and even needed, but Tiffany's upbringing did not seem to allow her to feel these things or even acknowledge them out loud. Then along came Larry and Stephanie and the wreck on the mountain that changed all of their lives forever... mystery, intrigue, laughter and even love...love in many ways. A real page-turner read on and find out what happens next but be careful it just may make you blush along the way.*

*Ms.Chatelain has given us a story to make us laugh and cry and even learn a bit about ourselves. Read and enjoy!!*

Written By:

Tonya L.

Chatelain

2002

Hello and thank you for taking the time to read one of my stories. I think of myself as a storyteller rather than just a writer. I tell the stories that are inside my head just waiting to get out. I want to take this time to thank one of the great people in my life. Thank you Cindy for all the hard work and time you have put into helping me and encouraging me as well as believing in me. You are my personal editor, my assistant as well as one of my best friends and much more. I also especially want to thank my children; Wayne and Courtney for being the best and greatest kids, if not a little ornery also, smile, that I could ever ask for. Larry you are the one stable in my life I can always count on. A special Thank You goes out to Cindi G. for your help and support. Last, but certainly not least. Ellen, Thank you for being my best friend and inspiration. Your love of books and reading is truly unique as are you. Ich liebe Dich Meine Freundin I love all you guys with all that I am.

# CHAPTER 1

As Michael was running his hands down Tiff's back she knew something was wrong. For the last five years she had stayed clear of all contact with guys, well, ever since her fifteenth birthday party anyway. Where she and her friends were sitting on the floor in the basement playing spin the bottle. That was what they had decided to do after her parents went upstairs to watch TV, leaving them alone downstairs to play nice as they had said.

It was Randy's turn and Tiffany had her fingers crossed that the bottle would point to her. She had this enormous crush on Randy ever since the sixth grade, she felt she would die if Courtney or Heather either one got to go to the laundry room with him for the... SHHH... KISS.

She held her breath watching closely as Randy's hand grabbed the neck of the bottle and let it spin. "Please, please, please!" she whispered to herself. As it came to a stop, she knew she was going to burst. "OH MY GOD!" she thought. "It did stop on me. I have waited on this day for almost three years, and now it is here and....OH GOD, I feel like I am going to be sick." Trying to play it cool, she watched him to see what he would do next. "Oh no, what if he is so grossed out by me that he won't even go in there? I would just die of embarrassment," she thought.

1

Now she was really holding her breath, pleading to herself, waiting to see if he would reach for her hand, at about that time he looked at her and grinned. She was, for a moment, relieved that he was going to pick her, then he did what every teen girl hates, he looked over at his buddies, winked with that stupid cocky, "I'm cool and going to get me some," grin as he grabbed her hand and almost drug her into the laundry room.

"My first kiss and with the boy I have dreamed about so many times. How lucky can someone get? Wow what a birthday! This was way better than any presents I had gotten and just when I thought the party had been a bust," she thought. As he shut the door and turned out the light they sort of just stood there. No one was making a move. "Shoot," Tiffany thought, "is this what they do, just come in here and stand, only pretending to kiss? Heck no, I did not dream about this boy for two almost three years to just stand here. Well are you going to kiss me or what?" she asked. Trying to sound like she knew what she was doing.

It was about then that Randy started snickering crudely. All the while Tiffany could feel her face turning red. He is laughing at me. He knows I have no experience and is making fun of me. "I didn't fool him," she thought.

"If we're going to kiss lets get it over with," Tiffany snapped, "or I'm going to go back out there, and don't you just know I will tell them you chickened out of a little old kiss," she said it with such determination in her voice that

2

she knew he believed her, while trying to be cool also. No way was Tiffany letting this jerk know she was hurt. About that time he grabbed at her arm and missed. It was dark in there and he grabbed her breast instead. At least she hoped he had been going for her arm. He dropped his hand and it was then she realized he was getting closer to her. Tiffany had not until that very minute realized how bad sweating boys smelled, and his breath stunk even worse, "NASTY!!" she thought.

"Stop it Tiff," she told herself, "you're just hurt and nervous, and it can't be that bad now can it?" She felt his breath moving in closer now and heard his mouth making those little sucking, clicking noises, It was like when you need a drink real bad and you're trying to collect spit in your mouth. In the dark it sounded even louder, "How gross!" she thought. "Heck Mom was right; I am not ready for any of this. Of course I would never let Mom know I agreed with her about this or anything else, for that matter." As an only child Tiffany felt it was her duty and responsibility to make sure her parents had a defiant child on their hands, so of course they would never want another kid. This would leave more for her from them in life. "Damn her for being right," she thought.

Just as his mouth got to hers, she turned her head, right in time to get a cheek and ear full of tongue and spit.

"Gross!"

3

"What did you say?" he challenged as he jerked his head back.

"Oh shoot, did I say that out loud" she wondered? This seemed to piss him off. He grabbed Tiff's arm to make her hold still. As his mouth reached hers, she was trying to pull away and say stop at about the same time that his tongue made its rounds again. He was making sure he got it right this time or at least his version of right. Trying to push him away, wasn't working at all either. Thank goodness, about that time Courtney started knocking on the door telling them to get out. Saying we had been in there long enough; it was her turn to spin.

Randy put his tongue back in its holder and snickered.

"Wadn't that bad, now was it? It was all your fault the first time anyway, you just made me mess up, that's all," Randy said. With that, he opened the door and walked out to the cheers of his buddies with a big cocky grin on his face.

"I waited and dreamed all this time for that??? GROSS, GROSS, GROSS!" Tiff thought as she walked back to the game, hurt, disappointed, and really grossed out.

Tiff was relieved that Courtney was the last one left to spin, because that meant the boys would soon have to go home. The girls were going to sleep over. Tiff really wanted to talk to them about what happened and how she felt about what went on in the laundry room with Randy. Knowing she would not have the nerve to tell them anyway, she was just relieved that the boys were going to be gone.

Tiff knew as Courtney spun the bottle she was so hoping it would land on Wolfgang. She had told her that she had a crush on him for a long, long time.

As it stopped all anyone heard was Heather saying "Oh yeahhh!!" with a huge shit-eating grin on her face.

"No way," Courtney said. "I want a do over now," she emphasized by grabbing the bottle again.

"Nope, you got to go with who it stopped on," Wolfgang said. Courtney stuck her tongue out at him, and then said. "Oh yeah, like if one of you boys spun it and it landed on another boy there's no way you would have went in there with him."

"Well that's different, we like to think of two girls kissing anyway," Scott said to the cheers of the boys.

Courtney just stared at him before getting up. "I'm not grabbing your hand either," she said to Heather over her shoulder as she stomped and pouted off to the laundry room. Heather was all happy as she ran to catch up to her.

As they shut the door Tiff heard Randy ask Scott, "Do you think they will kiss?"

"Get out of here man, ain't no way Courtney is kissing a girl, she's in love with Wolfgaaaang," he said slowly to jab at Wolfgang.

"She's kool," Wolfgang said. "Shut up and leave her alone Scott."

Tiff was still sitting there trying to get the nasty taste out of her mouth with some of the chips and soda her Mom had brought down to them. Then she started wondering how long they had been in there, it seemed like it had been forever. "I hope ours didn't seem so long, I'd just die if anyone thought we had did anything else other than kiss. The kiss had been bad enough and Tiff now wouldn't put it past Randy to make up a bunch of lies, She decided to ask Courtney how long they were in there, later when the guys go home," she thought.

About that time the door opened and out they came. "I wish I could have watched," Randy snickered.

"Shut up Randy, you're so immature," Tiff said. "Man, how wrong could someone be about someone else?" she thought.

That was five years ago and Tiff still never got over how much of a jerk he was. One thing that never left her mind for long, although she never knew why, was the thought of Heather and Courtney kissing. They never said if they did for real. Heather said Courtney had made her swear she would never say either way, and Tiff would never have believed she could have kept from telling it. Heather had the biggest mouth of them all growing up, but she had kept her word.

"Why did it make me wonder so much?" Tiff thought. "So what if they did kiss?" They all knew Heather liked both boys and girls, they just didn't know it had a name back then. It was never any big deal for them growing up. I think all it did was make the girls wonder about it and probably just made the boy's daydreams a little more interesting. When Tiffany thought about it, it didn't gross her out nearly as much as the kiss with Randy had.

# CHAPTER 2

Tiff had all but put it out of her head over the years. In fact, she hadn't thought about it at all in the last few months, not since this cute boy named Michael transferred to Baylor campus, where she also attended school. She never could figure out why it still lingered in her mind anyway after all this time.

From what Tiff heard others say this new guy had never been to Texas before. He was from California. When he won the USGA Amateur championship Golf Title and was offered a full ride here for his last year he took it. He was a senior and she a junior. Tiffany got his name from a friend of hers the first day she saw him. He was really the first boy since Randy that Tiff even thought about. "It has got to be different with him; it has been five years after all and I'm all grown up," she thought.

Tiffany noticed him the first week he was in her class. He was only in her Psych class but that was enough for her to notice him. At one point she even thought she had caught him looking at her a time or two. "I am sure it took him longer to know who I was though," she thought. He had so many friends right off they all just seemed to flock to him, boys and girls. Tiff envied that in him, as it was so hard for her to make new friends. It had always been that way too.

He had such ease with making friends and with all he did, or so it seemed.

Last Friday at the big football game while Tiffany was there alone, Michael had startled her when he came running up to her. Out of the blue he asked her if she wanted to go to the burger joint with him the following Friday. Taken aback and not knowing what else to say she answered with a very intelligent, "Sure," boy didn't she feel like a dweeb.

"O.K. then. I'll pick you up at 6:00," he said, smiling. It was about then that his buddies started blowing the horn and screaming out of the windows, so with a wave of his hand he ran off to catch up to his ride.

Tiffany had a whole week to think and worry about the upcoming date. "My first real date ever," she kept saying to herself and freaking out even worse. "At this rate I am going to have nothing but a face full of zits from stress," she told Brittany as they were looking through her closet full of nothing to wear.

"What am I going to wear? I have a whole closet full of clothing and nothing at all looks good on me right now. Brittany please help me! DANG, it looked cute last week, why not now?" Tiff said aloud to her mirror.

"First, chill out woman, we will find you something to wear that makes you look drop-dead gorgeous. Not that you need any help in that way," Brittany added more to herself, but Tiffany had heard her.

Tiffany sort of looked at Brittany out of the corner of her eye when she made that comment, thinking back on Heather and Courtney again before putting it out of her mind. Deciding Brittany was no help in picking clothing out, she decided to go shopping.

Brittany had only been Tiff's roommate for the last three months. It had been so sudden she didn't really know how it all happened, or why Brit picked her. All she knew is someone got pregnant and Brittany needed a roommate. Tiffany was about the only one who didn't share a room with anyone so when Brittany asked, she said yes.

The week flew by and it was now less than two hours to go before he arrived and Brit would not get out of the bathroom so Tiff could shower. As she reached for the phone to call Candy to see if she could use her shower there was a knock at the door. Looking at her watch she wondered who that could be. "Brittany, there is someone at the door, are you here?"

"No," she yelled back from the bathroom.

Opening the door her mouth flew open. "Michael..." she said in a stutter. "I... I... What are you doing here so early? It isn't eight yet."

"Eight?" He said, "No, I think there was a mix up. I am sure I said six p.m."

"No, no, no," Tiff said, "I remember you said that you would pick me up at... OK, I remember now.... Damn it... I cannot believe I messed the time up, I'm not even close to being ready."

He was laughing in a nice soft way, "Its ok...you look fine, just go like that."

She laughed as she looked down at her ragged shorts and her hairy legs. She was wearing a tee shirt with no bra, flip-flops, and to top it all off, she hadn't had a shower.

"Come on, you look great," he said.

Tiffany glanced over to the nice NEW outfit she had laying on the bed, waiting for her to put on when she got out of the shower. "What the hell? Lets go," she said with a scowl on her face. "We're going now Brit, no need to hurry your bath... have a nice evening online," Tiff called out to the bathroom door.

As they waited for the elevator, and all the way down to the lobby, Michael had his arm around her waist. Tiff wasn't comfortable with this at all, as there had not been more than twelve words between them since they met. Feeling very uneasy about his arm being around her she brushed it off as just nerves and went with it.

Most of the way to Sonic they didn't say anything. Tiff was wondering what to say and she was also wondering why Michael had even bothered to ask her out. He didn't seem to have anything to talk about with her, and come to think of it, they didn't even know each other very well at all. While they were eating, they tried to chitchat, but had little success at it.

After they finished he suggested a walk around the pond. Everyone knew about the pond. She also knew she was the only one that went there just to sit or read, everyone else went to make out. Tiff didn't care because she loved the pond. It was so quiet and peaceful and right down the hill from her dorm. "Sounds great," Tiff said.

Pulling up to the small parking area by the pond, Michael reached out and grabbed her hand as she was reaching for the door handle. "Hold on," he said. "Tiff, I have been watching you for a couple of weeks now. I have wanted to ask you out, but I didn't dare with what everyone was saying about you and all, now I am glad I did. You seem very..."

"Wait a minute," Tiffany interrupted, "saying? What are they saying about me and who are THEY?" Tiff said puzzled.

"Well I just didn't want to get turned down by...a..."

"By a what?" Tiff asked.

"Nothing, never mind, just forget it. Sorry I brought it up, let's just go for a walk," Michael said frustrated because he could not say the words he wanted to.

For the life of her, she could not finish the sentence that he was trying to say and not from the lack of trying. All the way down to the pond and half way around she thought of nothing else. She had to know what he was talking about; she couldn't take it any longer.

"Michael?? What were you trying to say before when we were in the truck? Please finish, you have me worried now. You said you didn't want to get turned down by a... Turned down by a what?"

Michael hesitated for a moment before answering her. "Tiff, I don't want to upset you but there is a rumor going around campus that you are a... a lesbian."

"A WHAT??" Tiffany loudly interrupted. "How in the hell would anyone think me a... a... one of them?" she finally got out in a hurt angry stutter. By this time she was very upset and on the verge of tears. How could someone, anyone say that about HER no less. "I have never even had a date with a man until tonight," she said loudly not caring who could hear her, "let alone with a girl."

"I know, that's all part of it," he said. "Well, that and the fact that Brittany is your roommate," he finished.

"Brit? What does she have to do with any of this? Did she tell someone I am one of those type of people?" Tiff asked a bit louder, feeling people starting to look at them but not caring.

"Then you really don't know," Michael said.

"Know what?"

"Brittany is a lesbian...she does not try to hide it at all ... everyone knows. How have you been her roommate all this time and not known? Did you not ever wonder why she does not date guys?? If it eases your mind to know, she never told anyone you were a lesbian. She just doesn't hide that she's one."

"Brit goes out all the time," Tiffany said, very irritated now. "She went out last night with...Susan. Well, they just went to a rally on...Oh...well, no biggie, they're best friends. They spend all their time together.... and," Tiff stopped in mid sentence and said, "damn it, I see what you mean. I just can't believe she is gay," she whispered. "But why would I think it strange that she never went out much, as I didn't date either? I cannot believe I didn't see it. Why has she not said anything to me? I don't understand this, are you sure she is one of "THEM"? We're not the best of friends but..." Tiff left it hanging in the air. "It doesn't make any sense ... why would they think that of me? I am not one of them," she was saying it more as reassurance to herself than to anyone else.

When Michael put his arms around her to pull her close; she fought the urge to pull away. She didn't know if it was from feeling cold or upset, but she was shaking.

"Here let me warm you," Michael whispered in her ear. "I'm sorry, I didn't mean to upset you," he said.

As he started kissing her neck and ear she just stood there afraid. "If she pulled away would he then think her a lezbo after all? And if she didn't pull away, maybe just maybe, he would tell his friends about it, and she would no longer be thought of as something like that...Oh My God what am I thinking?" she thought.

14

As Michael was running his hands down her back, she knew something was wrong. She did not like this; he was moving way to fast for her. "Stop Michael," Tiffany said as she pulled away. "This is going way to fast for me."

In the back of her mind, she wondered if he was the patsy boy sent by his friends to check her out to see if she was one of "THEM".

"Hey it's kool," Michael said, pulling away just a bit. "You OK?" he asked.

"Yeah," Tiff said. "I am just a bit chilly. It has been a long day, and well, I guess I am still a bit in shock about what we were talking about before. Do you mind if we head back and maybe meet up again another time?"

"Sure, that will be fine I guess," then he said seeing the look on her face, "no really, that will be fine, I don't mind, another time then."

The walk back to the truck was quiet, as was the ride to her dorm. "I'll walk you up," he offered, trying to be nice.

"It's early, I'll be fine, thanks anyway," Tiff said with a wave of her hand as she quickly got out of the truck. "See ya around."

"I'll call you tomorrow," she heard him say as she went in the door. She didn't turn around; she didn't want him to see the tears.

All the way up in the elevator Tiff could not stop thinking about what Michael had said. She was trying to figure out what bothered her about it so much.

Brit looked up in surprise as Tiff came into the room. "What's up Tiff? Is anything wrong? You're back so early, I didn't expect you for hours yet, if at all," Brit said with a wink of her eye. Tiff didn't say anything as she rolled her eyes at Brittany's little joke. She walked into the bathroom and slammed the door.

"Damn her and the horse she road in on," Brit said to herself, "she is in one of her primadonna moods yet again." At times she wished she could open up to Tiff and be close to her. She had had that closeness with her previous roommate, Marie, at least for a while anyway. She knew Tiff was a good person. After all, you cannot blame someone for the way they were raised but Brit didn't think it was an excuse either; she was in a catch-22 where it concerned Tiff.

Tiff shut the potty lid and sat down. "I can't stay in here all night," she thought. "But how can I go out there and face Brittany? After what all I now know?"

After about an hour in the bathroom, Tiffany, hearing no more sounds in the other room, opened the door slowly to see if Brit was asleep. Feeling relieved that she seemed to be, Tiff crept to the bottom bunk and got under the covers. Feeling a little foolish (as she tucked the cover around her tightly), because it was already hot in the room, she laughed to herself, "Get a grip girl, it isn't like she is going to come down here and attack you or anything." With that thought,

16

she threw the covers to the end of the bed as she did each night and rolled over and went off to sleep.

# CHAPTER 3

For the next three weeks every time the phone would ring Tiff refused to pick it up, to Brittany this was getting old quickly, she didn't like to answer the phone either. With no answering machine someone had to answer it or it would just keep on ringing and ringing.

Just then the ringing of the phone interrupted Brit's thoughts and irritated her once again. "Who is it?" Brit said into the phone. "No Michael, for the gizzlanth time she isn't here..." then she added in a snide tone, "she isn't here standing right by the bathroom door glaring at me right now!" and with that she slammed down the phone.

"What did you go and do that for?" Tiffany asked a bit peeved at what Brittany had just done.

"Tiff, what ever your problem is with him just tell him or end it and get over it. Damn this is so old now. You had one date with him, only one. He is still calling and you just ignore him. Did he do anything to you? Why are you acting like this towards him? You even walk around here as if you have a chip on your shoulder. Can't you at least talk to him to tell him to stop calling and coming by all the time. When he comes by you make me lie to him and say you're out. He's no dummy Tiffany. I am sure he knows it is all a lie. Even in class you refuse to look at him. Do you want to tell

18

me what is really going on? What did he do to you? Talk to me please!"

Tiffany just sat there looking at Brittany. She wanted to talk to her and tell her what Michael had said. He had put all new thoughts in her head or at least ones he had awakened from her past. Maybe the kiss between Heather and Courtney was what still made her wonder. She didn't know, she didn't know what any of it meant, but she knew she wanted to talk it over with Brittany. She also wanted to tell her about the dreams she was having almost every night since Michael had put the thoughts in her head, (she was sure this was the only reason for the dreams). She wanted to open up to Brit and ask her what it all meant. Tiff knew if anyone could help answer her question Brittany probably could. No matter how much she tried, the words just didn't come out. So she just shrugged at Brittany and said nothing at all.

"Whatever, I give up!!! Brittany said in frustration as she went out the door, slamming it loudly behind her.

Brittany was so mad at Tiffany. All the way to Susan's apartment she was cursing her out. She tried to calm down before she got there but to no avail. She knew every time she talked about Tiffany, Susan seemed to get a little jealous so she didn't want to go in there all mad and upset.

"You know what Susan?" Brittany said later that evening, "I am thinking about trying to get another roommate after the summer break is over."

"What?" Susan said, shocked. "Why? I thought you said she was easy to get along with and didn't sneak boys in all the time.... and that she was someone you could cheat off of from time to time," Susan said with a laugh. "OK, so she is a rich spoiled brat but other than that small fact she sounds ideal, and she sure is cute to boot," Susan said a little too wishful, then laughed.

"Stop," Brit said. "I mean it... she sulks all the time and I don't even know why she won't tell me anything. At first I thought that Michael dude that she went out with had done something to her. To tell you the truth, if he had I was ready to kick his ass, but then she just lets him keep calling and coming by. She won't even talk to him to tell him to stop so I have no clue. I am so tired of it!"

"Oh I see," Susan said, a bit hurt.

"What is it?" Brittany asked. "Did I say something wrong?"

"It just seems as if you have taken more than a roommate interest in Tiff," Susan said in a low voice. "I know I have no ties to you as we have agreed to be only friends and to see other people and all, but..."

"Now Susan, don't even start... I said no such thing. I am not even interested in her in that way at all, and anyway she is straight," even as Brittany said it she didn't believe it. She knew she was interested in Tiffany in a lot of ways, and for some reason she didn't care if she was straight or not. Why else had she got so pissed off when Tiffany came home upset and locked herself in the bathroom the night of her date with Michael? She had stayed in there for an hour and wouldn't come out until Brittany pretended she was asleep? This had puzzled her for a few days.... and to tell the truth it still does. She had never allowed herself to fall for a straight girl before, EVER. Marie didn't count she thought. Was that what she was doing she wondered? Falling for Tiffany??

"I got to run," Susan said. "I'll see ya later at the support group meeting."

"I don't think I am going to go this time," Brittany said, perplexed with her own thoughts. "I'll catch you the next time Susan," she said as she walked out the door.

It wasn't that Brittany didn't want to go to the meeting tonight...she did... but for some reason she didn't want to go with Susan. She had not wanted to spend as much time with Susan as of late.

"Hey Tiffany, I picked up some Chinese for us tonight, want some?" Brittany asked as she came into the dorm room.

"Sure. I've not had that in a long time. I thought you had that meeting tonight with Susan?"

"Nah, I decided not to go tonight, and anyway I wanted to say sorry about how I acted earlier. So this is a bribe, will you forgive me? What do you say?"

"All is forgiven if you tell me you got the Styx? You got to have them for Chinese food or it doesn't taste as good," Tiffany added with a chuckle.

"Yep, I got them," Brittany said. "But for all the good it will do, I have no clue how to use them."

"Here let me show you how to do that," she said smiling at Brittany as she watched her try a couple of times in vain. She got her Styx out of the bag and went to sit on her bed. "Come on," Tiffany said as she patted the bed next to where she was sitting. "It's easy, and if I don't show you I would feel so guilty if you go to China or somewhere like that and you end up starving to death. It would then be all my fault," Tiff said laughing.

For the next hour they talked and laughed until their sides hurt. More food ended up on the bed and floor than in their mouths. Both girls learned a lot, but not much on how to use the damn sticks, much to Brittany's dismay.

# CHAPTER 4

For the next three weeks Brittany and Tiffany seemed to grow closer. Tiff was opening up more and seemed so much happier. Brit was enjoying their new friendship and the closeness they now seemed to share.

The calls from Michael finally stopped. He was busy getting ready to graduate and she was pretty sure he was moving back home to California. Now that their junior year was coming to a close, Tiffany became sad. She didn't want to go back home for the summer and she had always wanted a house or apartment of her own. She knew she didn't want to stay alone. One evening when Brittany was chatting online as she did much of the time, Tiffany thought this was a good time to broach the subject.

"Brittany, have you ever given much thought to getting out of here and getting your own place?"

"You know I can't afford that Tiffany. I would love to, but I barely make tuition as it is."

"How about if we room together? You would save on your tuition since you would not be paying dorm fees," Tiffany interrupted, "it would be like now, except we could have a kitchen and no curfew... come on what do you say? Want to be my roommate again?"

"Well," Brittany started, "Susan has invited me to go with her to the Florida Keys to scout some jobs that she is looking at for next year and ...well, when were you thinking about doing all this Tiff? Tiffany?"

"What? Oh, sorry." Tiff said in a bitter tone. "Hey, no problem. You go off with HER and we'll just forget it all, it's ok..."

"Now wait a minute Tiffany, I am interested. I just need some information from you. Can you tell me like when you might want to start this? If I don't have time to go with her, I'll just tell her. She will understand I am sure."

"Why am I jealous?" Tiff wondered lost in thought for a minute as Brittany sat and watched her. "Why?" Seeing Brit watching her snapped her out of it. "Sorry, I guess my mind was else where," Tiff said. "OK then, let's talk," she tried to add in a light tone.

Brittany had decided not to go to the Keys with Susan. She didn't think it would leave her enough time to get every thing done, she just didn't know how she would tell her. She knew Susan would be pissed off at her, despite what she had lead Tiff to believe. But the decision made, she decided to give all her attention to Tiffany.

They had fun running all over town looking for places that summer. They got along so easy, joking, laughing, and just cutting up. For some reason they never seemed to get around to talking about personal things, growing up, their love life, or the lack of it.

As more time passed, Brit was sure that Tiffany didn't even know that she was a lesbian. If she did know, she was sure that she would never have accepted and embraced their friendship as fully as she did.

One evening as they were unpacking Brittany thought she would try to get on more of a personal level. Saying, "I thought I would let you know that Susan is no longer talking to me, for right now anyway. She will come around; it will just take her some time. She was mad that I didn't go spend the summer with her, and well, she is also upset that I moved in here with you," she added, "As I said before I am sure with time she will get over it."

"Why in the world would she be mad at that?" Tiffany asked. Then decided she didn't want to hear the answer because she wasn't ready to admit her feelings just yet for Brittany. She didn't think she was ready to hear what she was now all most sure Brittany would say to her about how she also felt. She wouldn't let Brittany answer (afraid of what she would say.) Tiffany moved on to some safe questions, such as, wanting to know how Brittany wanted to handle the cooking, cleaning and things such as that. She pretended that Brittany had said nothing.

"Around we go and I give up." Brittany said throwing her hands in the air. She got up and walked to her room, shaking her head.

Tiff pretended not to notice anything was wrong, or that there was stress between them. The whole summer went this way. They both did their own things, seeing each other only at home. They seemed to lose the closeness they were building, and Tiffany missed it more and more each day.

As the summer flew by, the dreams Tiffany was having became more intense and more frequent. She could not make out whom the person in the dream was, but she knew it was a new experience. It didn't seem like Michael and she knew it wasn't Randy. Since these were the only two men she had ever dreamed about, she didn't know who it might be. Maybe there was a new man on the horizon. Somehow in the back of her mind she didn't believe this. These dreams were more sensual, enticing, and even erotic in a way. She had felt none of that with either man, nothing even close.

Tiff promised herself she was going to talk the dreams over with Brittany soon. They felt almost as familiar to her as being around Brittany. She didn't know how, but she felt Brittany somehow held the key. She felt she might be ready to explore this with her one morning when she awoke after a very enticing dream. Summer was coming to a close, and school would be starting back soon. Tiffany knew she wanted what they had started building and even more.

"Hey Brittany," Tiffany said as she came out of the bathroom from taking her shower. "Later, when you get a minute, I want to run some things by you. Maybe we can have a good talk this time."

"K Tiffany, but it will need to wait until later this evening if that is ok. Susan called; she misses me and wants to make up. She also needs me to drive her to the Art gallery downtown, to pick out a piece of art from that new hot artist TLC before there all gone its for her friends birthday. She collects nudes of women and that is all TLC does. We should be back around 4:30 or 5:00 at the latest, want to talk then?"

"Sure, that will be fine," Tiff said, making sure no sarcasm could be heard trying to creep into her voice, also thinking it would give her more time to compose her thoughts. She would know exactly what she wanted to say to her, when they did talk.

"OK. I promise we will talk tonight," Brittany said with a smile and a twinkle in her eye that had not been there for most of the summer. She too was looking forward to a good talk. She had a few things she wanted to tell Tiffany also, feelings she was finding hard to hide as of late.

"I think I'll make spaghetti for dinner, do you think Susan will want to stay?" she yelled out to Brittany as she was headed out the door. "Damn," Tiff thought. "I guess she didn't hear me when Brittany didn't answer her back. I'll just make some extra in case." All the while hoping she would not need the extra at all.

# CHAPTER 5

Around 7:30 Tiffany was peeved; she kept looking at the clock every ten minutes growing more upset as the minutes ticked by. "Even if Brittany didn't know she was cooking dinner she did know they were going to talk this evening. She could have at least called to blow me off and not just stay away as it is getting very late." It was about that time that she heard a knock on the door. As Tiffany got up to answer the door, an uneasy feeling came over her seeing the two officers standing at the front door.

"Yes, may I help you?" Tiffany said to the two officers.

"Hello ma'am. Is this the home of Brittany Clemens?"

"Yes," Tiffany said. "She's my roommate. Why? Is something wrong?"

"Ma'am, may we come in and talk to you for a moment?"

"Sure, come on in," leading them in the door. Seeing the look on their faces Tiffany said, "Oh my God, is something wrong?"

"Ma'am, there's been an accident. A car swerved in front of a school bus and kept on going. As the bus overturned, Miss Clemens swerved hard to keep from hitting it. In doing so, she clipped the school bus wheel on the cars driver's side. Her passenger, as well as all the children and driver of the bus are shook up and in shock but they're all doing OK thanks to Miss Clemens quick reflexes. They are being checked out at the hospital and I am sure that they will be released soon."

"And Brittany?" Tiffany pleaded. "How is Brittany, will she be released soon also? Is she ok? Tell me she is ok," Tiffany pleaded.

"Ma'am, we want to make sure you understand that it wasn't her fault at all, but she didn't survive the accident. It happened so quick she never had a chance."

"Oh my God...Oh my God..." Tiff screamed. "We were just getting closer, and we were going to have a talk tonight. She promised me we would talk tonight... and... and.." Tiff was crying now and didn't even know that she was. "I didn't even get to say sorry for the way I acted these last two months," Tiffany sobbed.

"Ma'am, can we call someone to be here for you?"

"No, no thank you," Tiff said trying to dry her eyes and wipe her nose. "I'll be ok," she whispered, "I cannot believe this has happened. I can't believe she is really gone, just like that," she said to the back of her hand as she wiped her nose and sniffled.

After a few minutes of silence the officer said, "I hate to ask this right now but we need to contact the rest of her family and we need to get Ms. Clemens' parents information from you please."

"Did she feel any pain?" Tiff whispered.

"No ma'am. She went in an instant, she didn't feel anything, and she didn't suffer at all."

"I should feel better knowing this but I don't," Tiffany said.

"Ma'am, the passenger, Ms. Back is at the hospital. I think she will be released soon if you would like us to take you there to be with her we can?"

"Yes, thank you," Tiff said. Then thinking about it she shook her head and said, "No", as she walked to Brittany's desk to get the info they needed. "It is OK. I will go in my car so Susan will have a ride home. Thank you for stopping by to let me know. I think I need to wash my face before I go," Tiff said as she showed them out handing them the piece of paper with Brittany's home information written on it.

"Brittany's mother was so nice when she was here for a visit, maybe I should call her myself," Tiff thought, but she knew she would only fall apart again. "No, it would be better left up to someone else," Tiff thought, not thinking very clear at all. As she washed her face, she caught her reflection in the mirror. "What am I going to do? Why now?" she wondered.

Susan was sitting by the doors in a wheelchair when Tiffany got to the hospital. As Tiffany walked through the doors, they both started crying when they saw one another. Tiff didn't know Susan that well. She had only seen her briefly a few times, but she had always known she didn't much care for her.

Tiffany hugged Susan tight to help calm her down or maybe it was to help calm her own self down. After they both got a hold of themselves a little bit, Tiffany helped Susan get into the car and after getting in herself she could not make herself turn the key to start it.

"I blame myself," Susan suddenly said, more in a whisper than anything else. "It's my entire fault."

"What did you say?" Tiffany asked.

"We were fighting, arguing over you," Susan continued, "Maybe if we wasn't fighting she would have seen the accident in time to swerve out of the way, and maybe she would still be here," Susan sobbed.

"No, no, The police said there was no way to stop and that it wasn't anyone's fault except the car that swerved in front of the bus, the one that just kept on going. So don't blame yourself, Tiffany said," trying to comfort Susan between both their sobs now.

Tiffany wondered why they were arguing over her though, but she could not bring herself to ask. She didn't know what to say or how to say it when something like this happened. "You just don't say much," Tiff thought to herself. "It's late so why don't you just come to our house tonight Susan, and then we can figure out where to go from there."

By the time they got home, news had gotten around. There were forty-four messages on the filled up machine. Brittany was loved that was for sure. What surprised Tiffany even more was that over half the messages were for her,

31

people calling to check on her and to offer help and comfort. Nothing made her feel better though except the fact that Susan was there; she was someone Brittany knew well and somehow that made Tiff feel closer to Brit.

When she got to the message Brittany's mother had left she burst into tears again. She came back into the room and told Susan that Brittany's mother wanted them to know she had heard the news and that they were coming down to take her body back home. "She also asked us to keep all of her things, they could not face it right now and if we run across anything we think they might want to keep just send it to them. She also said to tell you when I see you that they send their love." Seeing Susan start crying again, she knew it was time for drinks.

Going to the kitchen, Tiffany came back with two hard drinks. She handed one to Susan just as Susan shook her head and said, "No thank you, I don't drink this stuff."

"Neither do I," Tiff said. "But right now we both need these." Looking at the amber liquor in the glass Susan started crying all over again. "Thank you she finally managed to get out."

# CHAPTER 6

After a long silence of drinking and crying, each lost in their own thoughts; Tiffany finally drank enough courage to talk about what was on her mind. "Susan, Brittany was very important to you in OTHER ways, other than just friends wasn't she?" Susan stared at Tiffany in shock, was she asking what Susan thought she was asking her? "Brittany had said Tiff had no idea that they were lesbians but somehow she had not believed her. No one could be that naïve," she had thought.

"I tell you what," Susan managed to slur out, "you tell me what you think Brittany and I were, and then, I'll tell you if you're right or wrong," Susan offered.

Silence again for a while and then Tiff said, "I think Brittany was a lesbian, and I was always hurt that she never opened up to me and talked to me about it. Did she think I would judge her? Or not want to be roommates with her or something. Did she really think me that bad a person that she could not share that with me?"

Susan was shocked to hear these words come out of Tiffany's mouth. "Somehow I knew you knew all along," Susan said. "Brit didn't think you knew. She thought she was saving you from something, somehow but from what, who knows?" she said with a shrug, "only she knows... knew," she corrected herself.

"Well I have not known all along. In fact it never even once crossed my mind that she was or could be until that night Michael and I went out and he told me that she was a lesbian. He thought I was one also because of rumors going around.... and well...I think for a while I was in shock and then...."

"So, is that what happened with Michael and you? Brittany had worried for the longest time that he had did something to you from the way you acted around him. She even said one night that she was about ready to kick his ass if he had hurt you."

"Brittany said that she would do that to him for me?" Tiffany asked dumbfounded. "If she said that then she must have really cared for me, and why didn't she tell me? All that lost wasted time for nothing," Tiffany cried.

"Yes Tiffany, she did say that. That was one reason we fought about you, jealousy. You know she was falling in love with you don't you? She said she was going to try and talk to you and tell you that night when you guys had your talk how she really felt. She knew you might kick her out or run away, but she said she had to let you know."

Tiffany was crying hard now, "I never knew she felt like that, and now it is all gone," she sobbed, "We will never get a chance."

Remembering they were talking about Michael, she answered Susan's question. "I don't really know what happened with him. I guess I am just... I don't know... I guess I just wasn't ready to date or something, but no he never did anything to me other than make me think."

As Tiff got up to get them refills for the fifth time, she decided to bring the whole bottle in with her this time. They drank for a long time and talked and cried and laughed and just sat staring at nothing.

Tiff didn't remember getting the blankets out of the bedroom or putting them on the floor. That is where they were when they awoke, well past 2:00 pm the next afternoon. The doorbell was ringing and they were both lying all over the living room floor with two splitting headaches to boot.

"Oh God, my head is killing me," Susan said as she sat up slowly.

"Yours ain't the only one," Tiffany said with what she could muster up of a smile as she went to the door. "OK, OK, I'm coming," Tiff said to the air, "stop ringing the damn doorbell."

"Tiffany, I heard the news," Michael said as Tiff opened the door. At about the same time, he saw Susan lying on the floor in only a tee shirt and underwear and Tiff in the same state of dress.

"Michael, hi, I thought you had went back west," Tiff said with surprise in her voice. Looking and feeling a bit embarrassed at the mess behind her and what he must be thinking about it all.

"That's obvious, judging from what I can see," Michael said as he looked around her to where Susan was on the floor in her underwear, "I was in town for the week and when I heard the news I had to come by to give my condolences in the loss of your friend," he finished after a long pause.

Then he turned around before Tiffany could say anything and walked away just like that.

The next few weeks, after the accident was over, things went pretty much the same way with them crying and drinking, doing the whole woe is me thing. Susan never went home, finally losing her apartment. Tiffany just sort of accepted her as the new roommate unofficially, and life went on like this, for a while anyway.

Susan came in half lit one night and pissed off, as was the standard most nights. Tiffany wasn't much better off herself most of the time. School had started and neither one even bothered to go to classes much of the time. If it had not been for Tiff's trust fund, they would be living on the streets. Neither of them bothered to even keep their jobs. Tiffany decided they needed to have a talk; she could no longer do this.

Before she could say anything Susan said, "Tiffany, we've got to get over this rough spot. Come on Tiff, we got to get back on track. Brittany would not want us to be unhappy like this all the time."

"I know Susan, I was just going to say the same thing, but how? How do we do that? All I think of is how fast it all goes, and how...how close I came to finding me... and...."

Susan didn't wait for her to finish. She leaned over and took Tiff's mouth. The kiss was one-sided at first but as it went on Tiffany found herself responding with a hunger in her she had not known before.

"I should say I am sorry," Susan said when it was over, "but I am not going to. I have wanted to kiss you for a long time. I always thought I was mad because Brittany moved in here with you and she never wanted to live in my apartment with me. But I think now it was because it was her here and not me, that's what I was mad about. Don't get me wrong I loved Brittany on so many levels, but Tiffany when I am around you, now, as well as before, it doesn't matter. I wanted you. I want to look at you and smell you and I want to kiss you. I know this is all new to you. I will not do it again if you do not want me to but I cannot sit and wait for the right time any longer, because we do not know if the right time will pass us by. I was pissed off tonight when I came in, not at you or anyone other than myself for that matter. I was pissed off because I wanted to tell you how I felt and to kiss you and I just didn't think I could, I didn't think I had the courage, but I am glad I did. Please just don't hate me. I know you think this is just because I am still hurting and I have said the same thing to myself but this isn't it. I use to dream about you long before all this happened with the accident. Tiffany do you hear me? Don't shut me out right now. Tiff?"

With that Tiff leaned over and kissed Susan. "I don't know what I am doing Susan," she finally whispered as she pulled back just a bit, "but I have butterflies and this electricity going through me that I have not had before, not with Randy, not with Michael, not with anyone. I don't know what it is or where it is from, but I want to kiss you again. I want you to kiss me...I want to..." nothing else was said as they were lost in each others lips, kissing with a hunger inside both of them.

It was at that moment that she knew what all the dreams had been about. She also knew who was in the dreams with her, she saw the person now as if she was awake in her own dream. She never saw a face or body but this felt like her dream... Susan was her dream... all along she had thought it was Brittany when she realized it was a woman and not a man in the dreams.

The dreams started after Michael had talked about Brittany. It was what he said about Brit and Susan that had started her subconscious working over time. She had not known it until that very kiss; there were no doubts now as she pulled Susan in closer to her.

# CHAPTER 7

At the risk of being clichéic, "the days following them getting closer seemed to be brighter," Tiff thought. Susan went back to work and school started going really well for them both again. Nothing went beyond the kissing at first; Tiff wanted to move slow and get use to the idea.

Susan knew that taking it slow was a good idea also. She saw what jumping in headfirst without thinking had done to Marie and Brittany. Brit fell for Marie from the first day she saw her. She could not believe her luck to get Marie for a roommate. She had seen her at the coffee shop on campus several times and knew her name and all about her, then when she saw Marie's name next to hers for rooms she knew she was in love, ok, lust but close enough for her.

Brittany knew Marie was straight but she also knew she was open and a big slut, Brit kept telling Susan that Marie was Bi not straight and what harm was there in helping her find her true self. Susan didn't feel it was as good of an idea as Brittany did, but no amount of bitching did any good so Susan sat back and let it play out. And boy did it ever play out.

As she sat and watched it unfold before her eyes. She was right, she knew it would burn out and she knew it would be bad when it did and it was very bad. It had almost drove

Brittany to the brink. Susan was afraid that she might not return from it if she went over. Marie did hop into bed with Brittany fairly quick, but she also hopped into bed with any man that came around and maybe even a few other women or so Susan had heard rumors to that fact. It tore Brittany to pieces.

All Susan would let herself do was be there to listen to Brit cry and bitch; she would not step in. She didn't think Tiffany ever knew how or why Brittany came to be her roommate in the middle of the term.... Brit never would admit anything was wrong. All she ever said was she needed a change because Marie kept sneaking boys in late at night and making noises to all hours; she said she just got tired of it.

Susan knew the real reason and she was proud of Brittany. Another woman not as strong would have not handled it as well. Try as she may, Brittany could never hide it from her. She knew Brit had to let it all go when Marie got pregnant and dropped out of school. The last thing anyone heard was that she was going to marry one of the men she had been with that she thought might be the baby's daddy. That was what made Brittany wake up finally, hurt and closed off, but she was going to be ok Susan thought. Brittany also now knew that straight and bi girls were unsafe on the heart. As all this ran through Susan's head she knew Tiffany was right; she did need to take it nice and slow.

One thing Susan did well was learning from others mistakes and although she didn't know what to make of Tiffany just yet, she didn't feel she was straight and she didn't feel she was bi. She wondered if she was just telling her self this to justify what she was feeling, but Susan did know that slow was how to go.

One thing that bothered Tiffany was that Susan seemed to have no family at all, and she would not talk about her past. Tiffany always wondered why. She felt that if she knew more about her that she might be able to open up to her more and take the next step, but Susan was adamant about never ever talking personal stuff when it came to growing up. Tiffany decided not to push her on the subject anymore.

They had been through so much the last few months and Susan knew she wanted Tiffany, she also knew she wanted it to last. She had never been in love like this before and she knew it was real. She had waited a long time for her and she knew she could and would wait as long as it took. A small voice in the back of her mind kept saying what if she is never ready for you? As Tiffany always hid the fact that they were together, not even any of her close friends knew. However, Susan knew she was willing to take whatever risk there was to be with Tiff.

They now found themselves sleeping in the same bed and Susan was finding it harder and harder not to press Tiffany for more than just kissing and cuddling. Just when

41

she didn't think she could take another night of lying next to her without touching her it happened. Tiff had said she had a headache and was going to go take a long bath. When she didn't come back into the living room after her bath, Susan became worried and went to see if she was ok. The lights were out except for some candles that flickered as Susan opened the door and there was music playing softly.

"Tiff," Susan whispered. "Are you awake?"

When Tiffany said nothing, Susan, assuming she was asleep, went to take a long bath herself. After she was done and feeling calm and a bit tired, Susan, being as quite as she could, climbed into bed trying not to wake Tiffany. When she was in the bed Tiff reach over and pulled Susan to her and began kissing her.

"I am so sorry honey. Did I wake you? I was trying to be as quiet as I could but I am a klutz as you know."

"No, no you didn't wake me at all. I was waiting on you. I want to hold you tonight, I want to touch you and have you touch me if that is ok? You sure do take long baths," she added with a smirk. "I thought I was going to end up falling asleep waiting for you to get out."

"Oh my God baby, of course it is ok. I have wanted so long to lay and hold you and touch you, but I was afraid you would feel like I was rushing you or putting you under pressure."

"Shh," Tiff said as she began kissing Susan. "I love you Susan, I love what we have. I am in love with you, I want

42

more. I feel very relaxed with you." Susan pulled Tiff into her, holding her tight. "Susan?" Tiff whispered. "I want to make love with you, I want to feel your hands and mouth on me.... Please baby make love to me."

Tiff didn't need to ask twice, as Susan pulled her nightshirt off and reached for Tiff's top, pulling it over her head. "You are so beautiful," Susan whispered. "I have wanted you for so long."

"I am scared," Tiff said. "I have never... not even with a guy."

"Shhh," Susan said. "I know."

Tiffany was more the aggressor. Susan was holding back a bit so as to not scare her with this being her first time and all, but Tiffany was having none of that. They spent the next couple of hours making love and then falling asleep in one another's arms.

Tiff had never felt so loved and relaxed with anyone and Susan was, for the first time that she can remember, very content.

Tiffany woke up early and just lay there; smiling and watching Susan sleep, playing with the bangs that fell over Susan's face. As Susan started stirring a little bit, Tiffany rolled over and kissed Susan, "Hey baby, morning, do you want some breakfast?"

"Oh, yes!" Susan said with a wicked smile on her face as she grabbed a hold of Tiffany rolling her over. Both girls giggled and then Susan kissed Tiffany's neck sending little chill bumps all over her.

"Oh, this is the breakfast you were talking about," Tiffany said as Susan's mouth found her nipple. "Damn that feels good," Tiffany groaned as Susan's mouth made a lingering trail down her stomach, she was making her way to her crotch and she could not keep from shivering, she knew from last night that she loved the feel of Susan's mouth and tongue on her and in her.

As they lay there after making love, Tiffany decided to ask Susan a question that she had been wondering about since last night and now even this morning.

"Susan," Tiffany began, "one reason it took me so long to get to this point with you, where we could do more than just kissing was because I didn't think I would have it in me to be able to give back to you what you would be giving me, if this makes any sense. I don't think I could ever put my mouth down... as she thought for a moment she finished, I don't think I could ever go down on you, like you do to me, will this bother you?"

Susan thought for a minute before she said. "Things take time, and there is always other ways for us to show our love and wanting for one another. I love the taste of a woman, so as long as you will let me I want to do that, I want to touch and taste you. But if you can't then you just can't; I will understand. I received so much pleasure from your hands and fingers and just from your caresses and hearing you moan, that is enough for me," she tried to reassure Tiffany, "and you sure knew what to do last night with your hands anyway. You're a quick study," she said trying to lighten the mood up a bit

# CHAPTER 8

For the next several months they were happy. One evening after dinner they were sitting on the porch drinking some raspberry ice tea and just watching the people that was out and about. It was a college town and most everyone on the street they lived on was college kids. "Watching them live their daily lives could be fun at times," Tiffany thought.

"My parents are coming for a visit in a week or two," Tiffany said, "and well, they don't know about... well you know... and, I don't want them to know Susan. I think you should move back to your room until they leave, they're old-fashioned and I know they wouldn't understand about us sleeping together or any of it for that matter."

Susan was hurt but she had expected it in a way, as Tiff would still not let anyone know about them. She even went to great links to hide it, from not sitting together on the days they had the same lunch, to not even talking to her when they ran into each other on campus.

"I understand Tiffany. I will not lie to you and say I am not hurt as I had hoped that our love would help you except it at least a little bit as we grew closer and that you would want others to know, but I do understand. I will not say anything to them or anyone else."

Seeing how hurt Susan was Tiffany said, "Honey, I don't mean to hurt you and if I have led you to believe we will always be together as a couple then I am sorry. You know I love being with you but I never promised we would always be together. My family and friends would just not understand and I cannot hurt them. Hell, I don't understand most of it myself, and I want marriage and kids one day later on. We are going to be teachers, and who would ever hire us if we live like that?" she said with sarcasms and maybe even a little disgust in her voice for the way they lived. "We are in college, when we graduate it will have to be different. We will be moving on from one another to our real lives and..."

Susan knew that Tiffany struggled with them as a couple a great deal but she didn't realized how much until now. "Stop it," Susan interrupted. "I don't want to think about it. We still have Christmas and then six more months after that to be together. (Also for me to change your mind, Susan thought) now lets not talk about it anymore right now, ok? Please."

Tiffany agreed. She pretended she didn't notice Susan slowly pulling away, Susan even spent a lot of time away during the time Tiffany's parents were there visiting. Susan told her it was to give them more family time together but Tiffany felt it was as if she was putting a wall up, to protect herself from getting hurt.

The visit with her parents went well and all; at least on the surface all was well. Tiffany could not figure out why her mother tried to talk about gay people several times though. She could not remember her mother ever even saying that word to her before. She even half wondered at one point if Susan had said something behind her back to them but she felt she knew Susan better than that.

Tiffany decided to brush it off as just a topic of conversation as it had been on TV a lot more now days, and her mother was a huge fan of the Ellen show. She still avoided her mother's questions and any eye contact with her when she was talking like that. Tiff was afraid that her mother some how could see it in her eyes. So she would change the subject each time, until her mother just finally gave up.

Susan was hurt. She tried not to let it show, but she dreaded each new day as it meant one day closer to Tiff moving on. Tiffany had told her she was moving to Colorado when she finished school, "that is if I get the job," she added with her fingers crossed.

Susan knew that was where Tiffany was from and she also knew it was a state she herself never wanted to see again. Tiffany said she wanted to move to the mountains and teach school there. Susan wanted to go to Florida and teach there. She had spent the last couple of summers scouting out different warm beach places. She hated the snow; it was a long lost, very bad memory for her. They had both always wanted to teach but that was where what they wanted to do the same, ended.

Susan decided she was not giving up on them or the future. She wanted to be with Tiffany; at least she was not giving up without a fight. She had been planning a little surprise for a few weeks for Tiffany; she had planned for it to take place Christmas morning. They were sitting on the floor opening presents they had gotten each other when suddenly Susan got up and ran to the bedroom saying, "Hold on I'll be right back, I have a surprise for you." When she was ready she called out to Tiffany telling her to shut her eyes. "Ok, you can open them now," she said coming into the room standing in front of Tiffany.

Tiffany giggled and said, "I feel like a kid." As she opened her eyes she saw Susan standing in front of her wearing a snowsuit, and coat and holding a small brightly wrapped box with a huge grin on her face.

Laughing, Tiff said, "What in the world are you doing girl? You have lost your mind not to mention you look totally stupid in that get up," she joked.

"Well here, open the box, then you will know what I am doing," Susan said, "and hurry before I burn up in all this, we are in Texas here as you know," she added, as she handed the box to Tiffany.

Tiff took the box and shook it. "What in the world is in here Susan? It's just a little too small for the snow skis I have wanted and been hinting at day in and day out for at

49

least the last month. Maybe you have a note hide in here as to where the skis are at," she added with a giggle thrown in.

"Just open it before I rip it open myself," Susan said growing impatient but she added with a smile, 'it is something you can wear, just not on your feet".

"Oh my!" Tiff said as she opened the box. "What is this for?" she demanded. "What have you gone and done? You have to ruin everything, why are you doing this to me? We had a deal Susan."

"Tiffany, I want us to be together, I love you and I want us to make a life together. I am not trying to do anything to you; I am trying to help you make us into an us. I am trying to show you that I am willing to adopt kids with you, if that is what you want or I will even move to Colorado to be with you. I will do and be what I need to for us to be together, I have the snowsuit all ready to pack up. And you can do the rest to keep me warm," Susan said with a laugh, trying to not notice the anger in Tiff's face. "Come on Tiffany, we are happy together and we love each other. We can do this together. We can handle the family and friends, Tiffany, please give us a chance I don't want to lose you baby. All my friends understood when I told them I was a lesbian. I know we can do this, I know we can together."

"Stop it," Tiff yelled. "Stop this now. We agreed, there is no you and I, there is no together once we graduate. Now stop it. I will not listen to any more of this nonsense. This was a college fling to me, and nothing more, do you hear me, nothing more. You mean nothing more than a fling to me."

With that Tiff ran out of the room, throwing the little box down that held the diamond ring and all of Susan's hopes and dreams in it.

"I never agreed to it. I never agreed to lose you," Susan said to herself as tear streamed down her face. "Never!"

# CHAPTER 9

The next six months were strained between them to say the least. Tiffany tried to make it fun like it had been before but their hearts weren't in it anymore. Susan was cold to her now and kept to herself most of the time. Tiffany heard from the job she had applied for in Colorado. Susan found out by over hearing her telling her mother on the phone one evening and was hurt that Tiffany didn't bother telling her about it first. All Tiffany said was, "I didn't tell you because I didn't want to hurt you again, as that is all I seem to be able to do now days," and then she walked out of the room as if none of it mattered anyway.

Susan knew Tiff was putting the wall up around her heart, and she could do nothing about it. She knew that she had also closed off her heart to Tiffany. They could not seem to go around it or even over it, so she just kept to herself. She got her own acceptance letter a couple of weeks later and started making her own plans to move to Florida when school was over. Tiffany seemed genuinely happy for her when Susan told her.

Tiffany said, "See I told you it would all work out for the best. Now we will each be doing what we wanted to do, and we get to live where we want to live."

Susan could not figure out how Tiffany could just turn her feelings off like that. "It sure as hell isn't working out the way I wanted it to," she thought.

As the last month together drew to a close, they began packing. It hit home for Susan that this was really it. The fact that she was going to lose Tiffany for good and didn't know how to stop it, it was like a bad dream that she could not wake up from. She didn't know how to deal with all this hurt that was inside her.

"Were going to stay in touch and still be friends ain't we? You know you're my best friend no matter what," Tiffany said, casually one evening, as if they were life long friends just going a different way in life for a bit after school. Tiffany walked into the room where Susan sat crying.

"What??" Susan said trying to hide her face as she wiped her eyes. "Sure, yea, friends... You know what I have an even better idea, why don't we just send e-mails to one another so to save on stamps and the cost of the phone bills and make it even more impersonal," with that Susan slammed out the door.

Tiffany knew Susan was hurting and angry. She had faith that she would get over it sooner or later, but this wasn't real life to Tiffany... life was after college not now, not like this and most definitely not with a woman for a life-mate. They had to go their own ways when it was over. "And go on is what they would do," she thought.

The day arrived when they had to say good-bye. The trucks had picked up their things the night before. All that was left was to get on the road, one heading one way and the other heading the other way.

"Tiffany, I love you and I always will," Susan said with tears in her eyes. "I don't want this and I am trying to understand as best I can why you do. I am trying to give you what you want. Please remember I am only a phone call away if you need or want me."

"I know you are," Tiffany said with a smile. "And ditto".

Having said that, Tiffany got into her car and with a wave of her hand out the window she was gone. No looking back, no nothing.

"Damn it," Susan thought, standing there stunned. "Ditto. She said bye with a ditto... not a hug... not even an, I love you... nothing but a damn ditto. What a cold hearted bitch," Susan thought. She knew Tiffany wasn't really that cold, or so she told herself. She just didn't know how she could act like this to her after all they had meant to one another.

Several years passed as they settled into their own lives. Tiffany wasn't far from Susan's mind most of the time. She tried calling her for a while, she even sent e-mails and wrote letters and cards. She wrote poems and she had even wanted to go visit Tiffany but Tiffany always said it wasn't a good time for her to come. Maybe later, it was always later... and later never came for Tiffany. After a while the calls all but stopped, Susan just sort of gave up with calling as well as all the other forms of contact. Susan felt bad about that but she never got any response at all so what else could she do but give up? Then one day out of the blue the phone rang.

Susan's heart about jumped out of her chest when she heard Tiffany's voice on the other end of the phone line. She knew it was her as soon as she said hello.

"Hey Susan, this is Tiffany."

"Yes, I know," Susan, stuttered out. "I do remember what you sound like. How have you been Tiffany?" she was trying to slow her breathing down and calm her nerves at the same time.

"Well I have been great and you, have you been doing good?"

Getting angry with Tiffany now because she was acting like the last several years had not even happened, "I'm just peachy," Susan said with as much sarcasm as she could muster.

After some more chitchatting from Tiffany, she dropped the bomb on Susan. "Susan I...I...I don't know how to say this... Well here goes, I'm getting married and I want you to be my maid of honor please," there was a long pause. "Susan, are you there???" Tiffany asked.

"I'm here," she whispered. Trying to understand why after all this time she would ask this of her. It has only been a few years, after all they had how could she have fallen for another woman and forgot her so easily. "Damn, she was cold," for after all she still thought of Tiffany all most daily. She often wondered what sort of teacher she had made or what she was doing at that minute in time. Sometimes at night when she was outside looking at the stars she would wonder if Tiffany was looking at the same ones, that somehow made her feel closer to Tiffany.

Susan could not even make herself pick anyone up at the bars for a one-night fling because Tiffany was still too much a part of her. Now, out of the blue, Tiffany has gone and gotten someone else and is marrying her just like that. "What the fuck?" she thought. "Tiffany, I don't know if... if I can," Susan stumbled all over her words and finally got them out.

"Come on Susan. Please do this for me, you can't say no. You know you're my best friend, I would never dream of asking anyone else and I love you to death. You will like Larry he is such a great g..."

"Wait a minute, what did you say?? Did you say Larry?? You're marrying a MAN??"

Laughing, Tiffany said, "Well yes of course I am marrying a man. What did you think??"

"I thought you were marrying a woman... they do that now days and it is even legal in some states."

The phone line was quiet for a minute before Tiffany said, "Susan, I have put that part of my life way behind me. It was just kids having fun in college. Please don't bring it up again. Ever!! I want you here with me on my special day. Will you please do this for me? I will pay for the plane ticket and everything." Susan could not believe she was standing here being hurt by this woman yet again and on the phone no less. Just hearing the words that Tiffany was saying was more than she could take, but she also knew she could not refuse Tiffany no matter how much she wanted to on this one. She thought this was so unfair of Tiffany to ask such a thing from her.

Knowing no way to get out of it she asked, "When and where?"

After taking down all the details Susan said, "Yes, I'll do it. I will be there the day of the wedding, but no sooner. I will take care of my own ticket and my hotel; I don't want anything from you," she then hung up the phone. Feeling empty and hurt and broken, Susan sat and cried over Tiffany yet again.

# CHAPTER 10

Tiffany could not seem to shake the emptiness she was feeling; she chalked it up to wedding jitters...after all she was getting married soon. She had tried to forget what she and Susan once had together. She knew she had to go on with her life. She thought that she may want kids, and the way to get kids was to get a husband and Larry was the sort of man any parent would want for their daughter. He was hard working and sweet; he would be a good husband and a great father. Tiffany did not dare tell him about Susan and herself, all he knows is that they were roommates in college and best friends. He was from Canton a small town in Ohio, and she knew he would not understand. He also knew her to be a virgin; to her she still was, after all she had never been with a man. He respected that and agreed to wait until they were married.

He knew she was very nervous about the wedding night so when she started acting distant several days before the wedding and before Susan arrived he dismissed it to her being upset about the "big wedding night".

Susan planned to stay in Colorado as little as she could, but when the only reservation she could get was over a week before the wedding she had to take it. She had decided to move on and put all thoughts about getting Tiffany back out of her head...but she knew she wasn't ready to get over her just like that. She knew to stay in the same town that Tiffany was in would not do her any good, so she made plans to stay up north of the Springs until the day before the wedding.

Susan loved the sand, the ocean and the city life. She had lived in Key West only a few years now but she knew it was home and she loved it, so when she stepped off the plane in Colorado to a snowstorm wearing only a thin jacket she was not happy to say the least. "How could anyone voluntarily live in such a state?" Susan wondered. She would have to remember to make sure her first question to Tiffany was why in the world she wanted to get married in weather like this, in the middle of the snow on top of Pikes Peak?

"What do you mean you don't have my Jeep?" Susan asked the sales girl that could have been no more than seventeen if that. "I reserved it weeks ago, and I called to confirm yesterday. I was assured then that it was here waiting for me."

"Sorry ma'am, but they're all gone now, last one went out this morning. I got a small Escort, you want it?"

"Escort?? Escort??" Susan yelled in frustration. "We have went around and around for twenty minutes. There is a damn blizzard out there and I don't think any damn Escort will get me to where I am going. Now get me a 4x4. How could you just let it go out this morning knowing I was going to pick it up today?"

"How was I to know you would show and besides my friend wanted it to go snow wheeling with. How am I suppose to give you something when I don't have one now to give?" she said as she chomped on her gum smacking loudly and played in her hair.

Susan could feel her face getting red, as she grew even madder. "I want to speak to your manager right now," Susan yelled between clamped teeth.

"She ain't here right now; if you come back next week when she gets back from vacation, you can talk to her then," she added with a smirk.

"Then get her on the phone," Susan said angrily. "I won't be in this damn town next week." She was trying to stay as calm as she could, all the while losing that battle with herself.

"Can't, phones are down. They've been down all day and will stay down for a couple of days I'm sure with the ice storm we're having and all. She wouldn't like me bothering her when she is on vacation anyway," she added.

At about that time a man walked in, "I need a vehicle Viv."

"Hey Norm. I don't have anything left but an Escort," looking at Susan she said, "Unless you're taking it."

"Give me the keys, the taxi's gone and I can't walk in this storm," she said with a huff. Signing the papers she grabbed the keys and went out the door. She could hear the man and the sales girls snickering behind her as she left.

Susan knew from the start that she was in trouble; she had never driven in snow or on ice before. Her cell phone had no signal and all the phones were down, so whom would she call anyway?? She was in a little Escort in the mountains; her flight to the little town she was going to stay at had been cancelled due to weather. She decided to take a small plane into another small rinky-dink town, west of her destination, and drive the rest of the way instead of waiting for another flight. She had a taxi take her to the rental place where she had a Jeep reserved. It just kept getting worse from there, as that seemed to be the only airport not snowed under she went with it, her first mistake. She had not bothered to try and call Tiffany to let her know she had decided to arrive several days early so she was out of luck for help from her.

Tiffany knew she would be arriving on the wedding day so she offered to help make arrangements as she was doing for all the guests that would be coming in for the wedding. Susan, not wanting to feel like just any other guest and not wanting Tiffany to do anything for her either, had told her she would handle it all and that she didn't want anything from her. She would want a car anyway so she would find her way to the chapel when she arrived. Her next mistake was agreeing to take this small car she thought to herself ... it was only around 4:00 pm but it seemed much later.

There wasn't a city in site and the snow was coming down harder now. She passed very few houses up in the mountains and not any with lights on. She became worried when another one of her spells hit her as she was driving. For months now she had been getting dizzy spells and had started losing weight slowly. At times even stomach cramps would hit her. She calmed down a little as it began to pass. She was getting a little unnerved when the defroster stopped working. Susan was trying to get it to work when the tires lost their grip on the pavement, and the car started to skid before sliding into the embankment. It came to a stop then sputtered before dying. "Hell fire, I was only doing three miles an hour as it was," she thought.

"Damn...damn...damn.... now what? No one would miss her for days yet, because they didn't know to expect her until then. The wedding wasn't until next Saturday and it was only Sunday evening." She had told Tiffany she would be there in time to meet her at the church Saturday even though she was only half joking at the time. Tiffany didn't know that; she had even seemed hurt when Susan had said it.

Not one house she passed the last hour had a light on. She knew from what the lady at the airport had said that most of the places up here were summer places and no one was there in the wintertime. She figured if worse came to worse she would break into one of them to stay, but she could not remember how far or when she saw the last one.

"Damn me and my big mouth," Susan thought. It was beginning to get really cold in the car now.

"Start, damn you, start," Susan screamed at the steering wheel. It would not even turn over now when she turned the key. "Damn, I have got to be the only butch that knows nothing at all about cars," Susan thought as she got out of the car to at least look under the hood. She found she couldn't even get the hood to open, and she had already traipsed through snow that came all most up to her waist to get to it.

"Well, that was stupid," she told herself as she got back in the cold car. Hitting her feet on the side of the car was doing no good either, she was trying to leave as much snow as she could outside, now wet and shivering and even colder.

She tried the key again, still nothing, not even a click... laughing in almost a cry. "Like me looking under the hood would have did any good anyway," she said aloud to herself. "Other than speeding up my freezing to death a little bit faster."

# CHAPTER 11

About an hour or more had passed when she thought she heard a sound. She couldn't make out if it was the wind or real. After a little while she knew it was real, but she didn't know what it was. She knew it was some sort of machine... and it seemed to be heading her way. About forty-five minutes later the sound stopped right outside the car. Holding her breath, she heard the snow crunching under someone's feet. Susan about jumped out of her skin when the knock on the window came. Susan tried the door handle but the door wouldn't budge now. It had only been about two hours since she had gotten back in the car but the door was frozen tight and she could not open it. She couldn't see out the frosted window at all.

"Hello in there, are you all right?"

"I can't open the door, It is froze solid," she called out to whoever was on the other side of the door, Susan was shocked to hear a woman's voice.

"I'll be right back, just hold tight for one minute. Don't go away," she said in a light tone.

"Funny," Susan said as she could hear the footsteps walk away then back again a few moments later.

"I'm back," the voice called. "When I say push... push on the door as hard as you can, got it?"

"Yeah I got it," Susan said. She could hear the metal binding as the woman with the sexy voice was prying on the door with something.

"Ok, push," the voice called. With that Susan pushed with all she had. Just then the door flew open and Susan found herself face to face with a black ski mask.

"Hi, I am Stephanie. You're one lucky woman. If I had not heard your car come over the mountain when I was out getting in my wood, you would have been stuck out here for days."

"Then I guess I should thank you for coming to my rescue. Hello, I'm Susan. How did you know I crashed?"

"It doesn't take a rocket scientist to figure that one out," Stephanie said. "You're in a little car on an icy mountain road, first I hear your engine and then just minutes more I don't. I knew you could not have gotten far in that amount of time. My Tractor could barely make it and it is made for this kind of weather, so I put two and two together, I get to find a pretty damsel in distress and I am now the hero," she added with a laugh. "Now come on before you stand here and freeze to death, we can talk at the house," with that she walked away leaving Susan standing there with her mouth open.

Susan hurried to catch up to her and was trying to stay close behind her newfound hero but was having a hard time keeping up. As she got to the Tractor, Stephanie was all ready aboard. Susan tried to climb up and slipped right back off the steps, landing on her butt.

"Are you OK?" Stephanie called over the noise of the tractor.

"Yes," Susan said, it was her pride that was hurt more so than her butt.

"Ok, lets try this again," She almost lost her footing again when she felt Stephanie's hand grab her arm, helping her the rest of the way up.

It was a long slow ride back half way up the mountain. Susan was frozen solid when they got to the cabin.

"What ever possessed you to go out in a blizzard like this and in a light weight coat not to mention that small ass car you have. What is it a Volkswagen or something?" Stephanie asked.

"It's a long story Stephanie," Susan said. "And it's not a bug it's an Escort, do you not know your car makes at all?" she teased.

"Please call me Steph, and you've got to admit that since it was pretty much snowed under when I got there I cannot be held accountable for not knowing the make of the car," she added with a laugh trying to lighten the mood. "Let me make us some hot cocoa and then you can tell me all about it," she added with a smile.

Going in the other room, Steph came back with some dry clothing for Susan to put on.

"These are not in fashion but they're dry at least," Steph said. "I am going to go change also; I'll be back in a few minutes."

As Susan told Stephanie the story over cocoa, she just sat listening to it shaking her head in disbelief.

"I am a writer and I come here to get away and write," Steph said. "But I don't know if I could have written anything as good as this story of yours," she said with a smile.

After they were all warmed up and in dry clothing and had finished the cocoa Susan said, "Thank you for everything but I've got to go. If you could point me in the direction of the nearest town and tell me how to get there, I would be very appreciative."

Laughing, Stephanie gave Susan the bad news.

"Sorry to tell you this my dear, but you will be going no where fast, not tonight and probably not for several days if this storm holds true. The lines are down and probably will be for a few days," seeing the look on Susan's face she added, "it isn't all bad. I won't bite, at least not until the fifth day," she said with a laugh, "and you do have a warm place to stay now. The phone lines do come on and go off several times during a storm so there is still hope yet, but you will not get a taxi or anyone else to get you to town from up here. They just don't come up here in this sort of weather. You're welcome to stay here and as I see it you have no other choice anyway. The next town is sixty-eight miles away. You would freeze to death on the tractor and as far as vehicles go that is all I have here. It took us almost an hour to get here from your car only four miles away. You're going to just need to buckle down and get comfy. I promise I will be a good girl," Steph said with a twinkle in her eyes, "At least I will try to be," she said laughing.

"I am sorry but I do not see what you think is so funny about all this," Susan said a bit peeved, "I don't have days to sit around up here on top of this mountain. I have got to get to the Springs."

"I'm sorry," Stephanie said, "but that is just the way it is, in the wintertime things move at a slow pace around here. That's why most people only stay up here in the summer time. The snow sort of sees to that," she added with a wink, "I thought you said you do not need to be there and wasn't even going to be there until Saturday anyway?"

Susan nodded her head to answer.

"Ok then," Steph said, "that gives us plenty of time to figure something out. Why don't you try and rest. We will see what the weather does and then we can plan from there in a few days?"

"Seeing as I have no other choice, I guess I will need to take you up on your offer," Susan answered. "Please don't get me wrong. I am grateful to you; I just seem to go from one mess to another is all."

"Sounds like I hear a pity party coming on," Steph said. "Get some rest tonight then tomorrow will look better. You have had a rough day. If you need me to I can tuck you in with a bedtime story," Steph said as she winked.

"Well then I will make sure I don't have a pity party," Susan said with a smile on her face, "and you better be careful making offers like that or I might take you up on the bedtime story," she said, hitting Steph with the small throw pillow that she had in her hands. She could tell that Stephanie was coming on to her a bit from the way she looked at her. For the first time in years she liked it, as she flirted right back without shame.

"Hey now, are you flirting with me young lady?" Steph said in an old ladies voice as she tried not to giggle. "Cause if you are you sweet young thing I think I like it."

They were both giggling now, "Ok, time for me to get some sleep cause it is getting pretty deep in here," Susan said, "and I'll be sleeping alone," she then added, "at least for tonight," she said with a wink then another fit of giggles.

As she lay there thinking she decided things sure were looking up after all, "they seemed a lot better than they had this time last night," she thought as she drifted off to sleep.

Tonya L. Chatelain

# CHAPTER 12

"I wonder why Susan is going to wait until the last minute to show up?" Tiffany said as she was talking to Larry. "I thought she was half joking when she said she would see me at the church Saturday. Dang it, what is up with her?" Tiffany thought. "Didn't she know how special a girls wedding day was? This was the day all little girls dream and plan for, and she has to go and pout on my day. Damn her."

"Well she may have had plans already," Larry offered, "you did sort of pop it on her out of the blue. I think it was nice of her to accept on such short notice, be glad she said yes. I got to run honey. We have tux fittings, but I will see you later for coffee right?" He kissed her cheek as she shook her head yes.

The wedding day was growing closer and this was the first time Tiffany had even allowed herself to think of the possibility that Susan would not even bother to show up after all. She had not called and from what she could find out from the airlines, they said they didn't even have any up coming reservation for her. They were booked solid for about another week due to the skiers.

"Damn her," Tiffany said aloud later, while she and her mother were busy making the little gift baskets for the wedding shower.

"What is it?" Her mother wanted to know. She could tell something had been bothering Tiffany for days. "Are you getting cold feet sweetie?"

"Oh, I'm so sorry Mom. No, it is nothing like that; I still have a bad habit of saying what I am thinking aloud. It's nothing, just worried about my maid of honor."

"Well honey, Susan is a lovely girl. She will be a great maid of honor. I am sure the dress will fit, you said she is still your size from what she told you on the phone," her mother finished.

"I know, I know," Tiff said. "I didn't mean I was worried in that way. She has not called and the airlines say she has no reservation, and... well I am getting worried. What if she doesn't show up at all? What will I do then Mom?"

"Well dear, I do not know Susan that well, but seems to me if she promised to be here then she will. We still have a week but I must say I was sort of surprised when you asked her to be in your wedding at all, then even more surprised when she said yes to being the maid of honor. I thought it would be too hard on her."

"Too hard on her, why would it be to hard on her?" Tiffany asked, puzzled. "It's my wedding day. What about it being hard on me?"

"Well knowing how she feels about you, or at least how she use to feel about you I was just surprised you asked her is all. I thought you might still have feelings for her as well," her mother replied.

71

Tiffany was shocked to hear her mother saying these things. "Mother, I want you to sit down here and talk to me about this? What makes you say these things?"

Tiffany had a sneaking suspicion that her mother knew, but how could that be she wondered.

"Dear," her mother began as she sat down next to Tiffany, "remember when we came to visit before Christmas, the year you two lived together?"

"Yes I remember," Tiff said.

"Well honey, I had sort of always thought you might be a lesbian. When I saw you and Susan together and saw the love she had for you, I knew it to be true. I saw you struggle with it and I even tried to bring it up a few times while we were there, but you would change the subject, so I thought that was your way of letting me know you didn't want to talk about it. I let it drop figuring that when you were ready to tell us talk about it you would come to me. When you never did I didn't know what to think. Do you remember?"

"No, I don't remember you wanting to talk about it with me," Tiffany said. "I do remember us getting on the subject of gays a couple of times but I never knew you were trying to talk to me about... oh my... I wish you had said something then, things may have been so different," Tiff said. She then paused before saying, "No, no I don't. I am glad you didn't say anything. I don't think I could have talked about it with you and Daddy anyway. I was so scared you would disown me, or something. Mom how did you know?"

"Well, I didn't really know for sure, it was just a feeling I had for a long time," her mother said. "I just sort of thought it to be true. My little brother is gay. Did you know that?" Her mother asked.

"Uncle Roger is gay?" Tiff said. "No, I didn't know that."

"Well he is and has always been. We always knew it; we just didn't talk about it much. One day when you first went off to college, Roger and I were talking about you. He said he thought you might be or that you were at least confused about it. I think maybe he knew even before you did. At first I brushed it off, but the more I thought about it the more I thought he might be right. Honey, I love you, you're my only baby and I was OK with you being a lesbian if that was what made you happy. I could never think badly about you no matter what. When you moved out here and she didn't move with you, I didn't understand why she didn't. I thought you two had a fight or something. I think, in my mind, I always expected you two to make up and she move here. As time went by and that didn't happen I just sort of put it out of my mind thinking I had been wrong, or that you would tell me when you felt I should know. Then a few years later, when you told me about Larry, I think I was in shock. I had always wanted grandchildren, but I had talked myself out of that possibility knowing what I thought I knew. All I was hoping for was that you and Susan or whomever you were with would want kids also and would adopt. I am not even sure I heard you say you and Larry were getting married at first it just didn't register at all."

Tiffany sat in shock listening to her mother talk; she didn't even feel like she knew this woman sitting by her right now. Hearing how she was talking so open and unguarded made Tiffany have more respect for her than she thought possible.

"Susan had said way back then that I should talk to you and tell you, that you would understand, but I just didn't believe her. I never thought you all would understand any of it, and I didn't want to be judged by my friend either. I did love her so Mom, I really did. I had feelings and emotions with her that I had never had before with anyone, but I knew my family came first. You always taught me family first and it stuck with me."

"Well honey," her mother said, "Susan was family, when you fall in love with someone they become part of the family. As for the friend's part, would they really be friends or the sort of friend you would want if they judge you? You said you loved her honey, how do you feel now? I know Larry is in the picture now and it had been several years? But do you still love her?"

In a whisper with tears in her eyes Tiffany said, "YES! I have not let myself think about it or her in all these years but yes, I do still love her and miss her, very much."

"Oh dear," she heard her mother say.

"Mom, I do think the world of Larry. He is so nice and I don't want to hurt him, but yes, I still love Susan."

"Larry is a great guy," her mother agreed, "he will be hurt but you have got to tell him, he deserves that. It isn't fair to him to not know the truth. If you plan on going through with the wedding he needs to know before so he can decide if that is what he wants in a wife. If you plan to call it off he needs to be told, it is only right honey. Doesn't he know about you and Susan?"

"No Mom. He knows she was my roommate and we are friends but nothing else. I could never bring myself to tell him or anyone. The sad part is I don't even know now why I felt I couldn't tell anyone. I've got to go Mom; I've got to go do a lot of thinking. Tell everyone I am sorry to miss the shower and I will be back later."

As she hurried to the door she stopped, turned around and ran back to her mother. "Thank you Mom. I love you so much," Tiffany said hugging her Mom for several seconds.

"Tiffany," her Mother said pushing her at arms length, "honey, no matter what, I mean no matter what, listen to your heart, it will know what the right thing to do is, then when you know what it is telling you to do, do it. I love you baby, no matter what."

# CHAPTER 13

Tiff went for a drive to clear her head; she knew the roads were bad. She had in the last few years gotten use to them being this way much of the time. She knew she would need to concentrate on her driving and not everything else so it would give her time to clear her head. When she got to her secluded spot, she got out of the Jeep and hiked to the big rock that perched out over the bluff over looking the Springs.

She loved this place, it was always able to sooth anything that was wrong with her but she had such an empty ache in her heart that she had her doubts this time. She knew only one person could fill it. She also wondered if it would be too late for her and Susan if this were what she even decided to do.

"What am I going to do?" Tiffany asked herself out loud. It had never occurred to her that she could have her family as well as Susan. Now she learns that her mother understands and still loves her? "How could this be? Where in the world have I been for all these years?" she wondered. She didn't feel like she knew her Mom at all now. Then there is Larry, sweet, sweet Larry. She knew she could not marry him just to keep from hurting him, she knew that would hurt more in the long run. She knew she was supposed to be Mrs. Larry Yarns in a few short days. Was it too late to pull out now? Family and friends had already started arriving.

Tiffany knew she was all messed up in her way of thinking. She needed Susan here to talk to; maybe Susan didn't even still love her. "She may not even still want me," Tiffany thought. She had not let herself think about it at all, so she didn't even know if it was still in Susan's voice when they talked the other day.

Maybe she had moved on and didn't love her anymore now and that is why she said yes to be my maid of honor. "Damn, too many questions," Tiffany thought. "If Susan didn't love her would it matter? Would she then go ahead and marry Larry?

Somehow she knew it didn't matter what Susan's answer would be, she would have to call it off. She just could not go through with it. I've got to go talk to Larry first thing, he deserves at least that much," she said to herself.

The drive was slow going as she headed back home and it was lunchtime when she got there. Larry had just arrived to have lunch with her.

"Larry, can we go talk please?" Tiffany asked.

"Honey, lunch is ready and everyone is here. Can this wait until after lunchtime?"

"NO, it can't Larry!" Tiffany snapped, seeing his face she added, "I'm sorry, I didn't mean to snap, we just really need to talk now. Let me tell Mom to go on with lunch. I'll be right back, don't go anywhere, please," she begged.

"Ok, Ok, I'll wait," he assured her.

"Mom, I am going to talk to Larry. Please have lunch with everyone, you were right; I am going to listen to my heart. If it is too late for Susan and I at least I will not make a mistake and hurt Larry even more. Thank you so much for the talk and your support, now I've got to go do this. Telling Larry is the hardest thing I have had to do, and I am scared, but it is only right that I do this." With that Tiffany walked out of the room, she did not see the proud smile her Mother had on her face.

The talk with Larry was hard for Tiffany, harder even than she thought it would be, explaining about Susan and college and about the wedding being off. He seemed to be in shock as he left when she had finished, without saying a word he just kept shaking his head. Tiffany was sorry for hurting him; she knew he would be ok. She hoped he would be anyway.

The phones came back on that afternoon for a bit before the snow started again. Tiffany spent all evening calling all the airlines and Susan's house a hundred times. She was very frustrated by dinner when she could not find her or any information on her.

Her mother helped her call everyone from their side of the family to let him or her know the wedding was off. Some were not happy to say the least as they had flown in from other states and were at hotels. With a storm like the one that was moving in they could be stuck there for days.

Tiff didn't know if she should call Larry's family or let him tell them, she tried to call him to find out what he wanted her to do but she got no answer from his house. As she let the phone ring in case he was asleep or in the shower her mind drifted back to when she first met him. It was at the park; she was there grading some paper's as she often liked to do and as luck had it so was he.

She had seen him there many times but not until today did she ever approach him. Today was different, she walked over and said hello and they hit it off. She liked the fact that he, too, was a teacher. He taught fifth grade and she taught eight at different schools. They had that to talk about as well as so much more they also liked to compare stories of the children.

The two of them had such ease about the way they got along and Tiffany felt protected as if she had an older brother. "Oh my God," she thought, not until that minute did she realize that is what she had felt for Larry. She had mistaken it for true love, "I have had blinders on for these last few years," Tiffany thought, hearing the phone still ringing in her ear she hung it up.

She decided to get her mothers advice as to if she should call his side or not, her mother suggested that they should at least go ahead and call Larry's parents and they could inform the rest of the guests if he didn't, or they would end up going to an empty church. They decided to let him fill them in on the particulars later, so Tiff called them after dinner.

# CHAPTER 14

They had a great day together. Susan decided the night before while she was laying on the couch trying to sleep, to just forget Tiffany and let what was going to happen with Stephanie or anyone just happen. Tiffany was gone; she was getting married to a man and had all but forgotten Susan. So be it, she thought as she drifted off to sleep.

She and Stephanie got along great and for once in years Susan had a smile on her face. Steph woke Susan early with the smell of bacon, ham, and eggs cooking in the kitchen.

"Wow that smells great," Susan said, walking up behind Stephanie. "I didn't realize how hungry I was until I woke to that smell."

"Good," Steph said. "I made a lot. I was counting on you being ravenous," she said with a bright smile. "Now eat up. You will need your strength."

"Oh no," Susan groaned. "I don't think I like the sounds of that, it sounds like you are going to be putting me to work."

"Your darn right I am... you didn't think you were going to get a mini vacation out of your little accident now did you?" Steph said with a laugh. "We're going to get in wood and shovel the long drive to start off with before we get hit with more snow. Now eat up my dear."

Susan was burning up about half way through the shoveling of the drive when she felt a big thug hit her, "What the..." laughing, she ducked just as Steph hurled another one at her.

"I'll get you back!" Susan called out as she ducked behind a tree. Scooping to grab some snow she got hit again...they pounded each other for a bit before collapsing in a heap on the ground in fits of laughter.

"Let's make snow angels," Steph said.

Looking confused, Susan asked what that was.

"You don't know what snow angels are? You must have lived a sheltered life," she teased as she lay on the ground with her arms and legs spread wide and started flapping them back and forth like crazy.

"My father was too strict to let us do this in the snow, he would have said the devil would get us if we did such a thing," Susan said with a hint of a smile, "and mom would have been mad that we were laying on the ground in our clothing, so I guess my life WAS a little sheltered."

"Now what are you doing?" Susan wanted to know as she watched Steph.

"Making snow angels silly, I told you already." Steph said. "Now it is your turn, lay down and try it."

"I know your making that," Susan said, "I was meaning what were you doing with your finger?"

"Oh, I was just drawing in the eyes and mouth. I like to make mine complete."

After they were finished, and as they stood looking down at the work of art they had made, they both burst out laughing. Susan's looked like a big bear had made her angel for her; it had no definition at all to it.

"Ok you win," She said, "yours looks much better, it looks like a real angel. I think I need a lot of practice but it is to dang hot to do anymore today. I am burning up, how can it be so cold here and me be so hot?"

"Let's go in before you catch your death," Steph said, it was getting near dinnertime anyway. After getting into dry clothing herself, she gave Susan a towel and some more dry clothes for her to put on.

"Go take a bath and I will make us some dinner," Steph said. As Susan swished off to the bathroom in her wet clothing, Steph started dinner. It was about that time that the phone rang.

"Hello," Steph said in a hushed tone. "Hi Rose...yes, I know...yes, I know...she is OK...she is here with me...no, no it is OK...How did you know about the wreck? I thought so... when did the phones come back on...OK, Hon its hard to hear you with all the crackling so I'll go love ya, thanks dear, bye." And with that she hung up. She wondered if Susan had heard the phone ring? She also wondered if Susan didn't hear it would she tell her it was back on?

"Dinner is done," she called to Susan who had drifted off to sleep in the tub.

83

"Thanks, I'm getting out," she called back. "I think I just fell asleep in your tub."

"That's ok," Steph said," I do it all the time."

At dinner Steph told Susan that Rose from up the road had called. She had wanted to tell me there had been an accident down the road a piece and wanted to also let me know the lines were back up but not for long, as they expected another nasty storm tonight.

"It is late. You will not be able to get a ride into town until tomorrow depending on the storm tonight. Even then, no telling if you will get anyone to take you the extra fifty miles to the Springs until Thursday. You're more than welcome to stay here as long as you need to," she heard herself say to Susan.

A flicker of worry crossed Susan's face but only for a minute then she said, "Thank you. I think I would like that."

"Good," Steph said with a smile. "Go sit and I will bring us some hot cocoa." As Steph made the cocoa Susan walked around the living room looking at stuff, when she got to Steph's desk she stopped, seeing her laptop open she leaned over to read a bit.

"Wow, this is great," she told Steph as she came in carrying the cups. "You didn't tell me you were this good."

"Thank you," Steph said a bit perplexed. "I don't let anyone read them until I am done, but you know what? I think I like it that you read some," she said with a smile.

84

"Good, I don't want you mad at me," Susan said, "but I couldn't help myself."

"Hey, how about I let you read some more," Steph offered.

"I would like that," So for the next couple hours she read, forgetting all about calling Tiffany to let her know she would not be there. Steph sat impatiently waiting for some sign that she liked it or didn't like it, anything, just so she would know. Finally Susan looked up, for a minute she said nothing, she just sat looking at Steph.

"Come on, come on before I start biting my nails," Steph said. "I can't stand this, this is why I do not let anyone read my stuff."

"Chill out," Susan said smiling. "It is good, I mean really, really good. Each page makes me want to read more. And believe you me it is hard for me to find a book that can hold my attention."

Steph felt proud with what Susan was saying. "Thank you." Steph was about to say more but decided not to, not yet anyway. As they sat watching the fire in the fireplace try to burn itself out and hearing the wind and snow whip around outside, Susan reached over and took Steph's hand in hers.

"Do you mind this?" Susan asked.

"No, not at all."

With that, Steph leaned over and kissed Susan soft and lightly. Susan kissed back with a hunger in her she had forgotten she had. Their kissing grew to a new intense level; thoughts of Tiff kept popping into Susan's head.

"Stop," Susan told herself. "That part of your life is over." Susan was beginning to feel again and she liked the feelings. She needed this it had been so long. She needed the closeness of another person and she really liked what she knew of Steph so far. She had not even let herself kiss another woman since...

"Damn it," Susan said pulling back.

"What is it?" Steph asked, a little confused. "Did I do something wrong?"

"No, no, not at all. I am sorry that this popped into my head right then; I didn't mean for it to, but I just forgot to call Tiffany and they are expecting me at the church in a few days... hell, I am the damn maid of honor. I've got to let them know I have decided to not go while the phone is up, or I may not get another chance," she added. "I know it is late but I've got to call and at least let them know I will not be there. I'm sorry," she added with another kiss.

"No need to apologize at all, but it will be a miracle if the phone lines are still up this late. It may also be hard to hear, as the lines are always bad this time of year. You might want to go into the hall where the popping from the fire doesn't bother you, and you will have more privacy also," Steph said with a smile.

# CHAPTER 15

Holding her breath as she picked up the phone receiver with a rush she exhaled loudly. There was still a dial tone, barely but one nonetheless. Her hands shook as she dialed the number, and as Tiffany's sleepy voice came over the staticy line, she caught her breath once again.

"Hello," Tiffany said.

"Tiff, this is Susan, I don't have long as these line are bad. But I wanted to let you know I cannot make the wedding. I'm sorry I know it's short notice, but I won't be there." Susan had already made up her mind to not tell her anything other than she wasn't going to be there.

There was silence on the other end so she didn't know if the line was still connected or not..."Hello are you there?" Susan asked.

"I'm here," Tiffany said. "I'm so glad you called I have been calling looking for you everywhere, because I've got something I need to tell you also..." after a short pause she went on, "there isn't going to be a wedding Susan. I called it off yesterday. I love you Susan. I have been such a fool and I realize that now. I love you and if you will have me I want you back. I am so sorry baby; I was really a fool. Do you think you will ever be able to forgive me? Baby? Baby?"

The line was dead. Tiffany didn't know at what part it went dead. She didn't know how much or how little Susan had heard.

"Hello? Hello? Dang it, the line went dead," Susan told Stephanie.

"At least you were able to get out that you wouldn't be there before the line went dead, didn't you?"

Susan was quite for a minute thinking about what she thought Tiffany had said before the line went dead. Was it possible that she really said she loved me? Susan wondered. She had waited years for her to say that she wanted her back. If she did call off her wedding for me, does it make a difference at all? Will I take her back? She knew just a few short days ago the answer would have been yes. Now she wasn't so sure.

"Oh yes, I let her know in time...she was saying something I could not quite make out. I know she said she called the wedding off, or at least I think that was what she said."

"Was that all she said?" Steph asked casually, trying not to pry but too curious not to ask.

Susan smiled at Steph. This woman had a pull on her all ready; she knew she wanted to see where it would lead. Taking Stephanie's hand, she walked with her to the bedroom. As they undressed, Susan could not get out of her head what she thought she had heard Tiffany say. Did she really say she loves her and wants her or did Susan just need Tiffany to say it so much that she just thought she heard it through all the static?

Susan brought her mind back to the kissing and Steph's hands searching her.

"Steph? I'm sorry honey I am just really tired, it is only midnight but I feel like it is at least 3:00 am. It has been a long day, and to tell you the truth my mind is elsewhere and this would not be fair to you. Do you mind if we just go to sleep?"

Stephanie was a bit hurt but only said, "I understand. I know that call threw you for a loop; it was nothing like you expected it to be. I know you weren't ready for what she said to you. Will you please sleep here with me though?"

"Yes," Susan said as she lay down and cuddled up to Steph, "I would like that very much," then she whispered, "it will get better I promise, just give me time."

She didn't know if she was saying it to reassure herself or Steph, but she needed to believe it would get better. She could not fall off to sleep right away, so she lay there trying to go back over the phone conversation in her mind.

"What did it mean?" Susan wondered. "If she did say she loves me does it change anything? After years, could I? Would I just forget all the hurt she has caused and take her back? And if I just wished she said it does it mean I'm not ready to move on and be with Stephanie?" Too many questions... too many questions without answers...

questions, I need to have answers for," was the last thought that Susan had as she finally drifted off to sleep.

Stephanie always found herself getting attached too soon and she always got hurt, somehow this one was different. She wrecked the car here for a reason, Stephanie thought, but for what reason? She knew Susan wasn't asleep lying next to her, and she knew she was thinking about Tiffany. She didn't know why she was feeling a bit jealous. She had only known this woman for two days, but she knew she liked her a lot already and didn't want her to get hurt again by Tiffany. She also knew she had no choice or say in any of this. All she could do was snuggle close to Susan and go to sleep. Time would tell, as Miss Rose always says.

Stephanie woke up to find the bed empty and cold next to her; it was still early morning and dark outside. (Thinking Susan went to the bathroom, she lay there for a few minutes listening to see if she could hear her stirring around, hearing nothing) After a bit she got up and went to the kitchen, then on into the living room. There on the couch she saw Susan lying sound asleep.

She had gotten up sometime after Stephanie had drifted off to sleep. Stephanie sat and looked at this woman that she didn't even know much about, as she slept with the moonlight filtering through the window, falling across her cheek. She knew she was already starting to care for her to the point that she knew if Susan went back to Tiffany her own heart was going to get hurt. With that thought still lingering in her head, she grabbed another cover off of the chair putting it over Susan to keep her warm from the chill that was in the air and went back to bed.

This time Stephanie woke up to the great smell of breakfast cooking. She got out of bed and went to the kitchen to investigate. Walking up behind Susan she put her arms around her waist and pulled her towards her.

"Good morning," she said in Susan's ear, kissing her neck. "I have not awaken to the smell of cooking since I was still living at home, and I must say I like it," she added with a smile.

"Good morning yourself," Susan said in her cheeriest morning voice, pulling away as she put on the pretense she was going to get a plate to put the eggs on. "You were so nice to cook for me yesterday morning; I thought I would return the favor." Susan knew telling Stephanie about what she had decided to do was going to be hard.

Feeling a little dejected Stephanie plastered a smile on her face. "I think I will go freshen up and dress, unless you need my help on anything," Steph said.

"I think I have everything under control," Susan said, relieved that she didn't have to talk about it right now.

Over breakfast Susan told Stephanie what she thought she might have heard Tiffany say.

"What does this mean for you and I?" Stephanie asked.

"I thought about that a lot last night," Susan said. "I finally went to sleep but not for long as I was so restless. I went to the couch early this morning so as not to wake you. I think I need to go to the Springs and talk with her; I need closure on all this either way. I do not know what it means for us, if she said it or if she didn't and I am not sure it matters either way. I will not know what it all means until I talk to her. Remember I have a lot of years of nothing but hurt from her, I can't and won't just forget that either, and you do play an important part in this whole thing now also," she added with a squeeze to Steph's hand. "So, please give me a few days to straighten this out. No matter the out come I will be back to let you know one way or the other."

"Ok, I understand," Stephanie said. "Ok," was about all she could say. "It looks as if it is going to be a nice day," Steph added. "I will take the tractor around to Miss Rose's and see if I can use her jeep four by four. If she lets me, I will get you to the Springs today my dear."

After breakfast, while they were clearing the table, Stephanie took hold of Susan's arm and turned her around. "Susan, I know we have only just begun. I think we both know it could be something wonderful and I want you to know my door is always open to you. I also want you to know that I will understand whatever you decide to do, but know I do care about you. Please don't get hurt again," then she leaned in for a long soft kiss, which Susan returned with new feelings for this woman.

Before Susan could say anything, Stephanie grabbed her coat and gloves and went out the door. Promising to be back in a bit.

# CHAPTER 16

Tiffany just could not make herself get out of bed; she hadn't gotten any sleep all night long. Thoughts of Susan filled her dreams when she tried to drift off. She had done her so wrong; how could she blame her for not even showing up for the wedding? How could she blame her at all; what had she been thinking in even asking her? She knew that was just it, she had not been thinking at all.

Her mother got to Tiffany's house bright and early, seeing that she was still asleep she let herself in and made coffee. When it was ready she took a cup into Tiffany's room, waking her to see if she needed anything.

"You know what mom? How that must have hurt Susan, to love me as much as she did and have me act like that to her back. Then to just threw her away as if she was nobody. Hell, I denied her the whole time we were together. Then, I just left her and moved away. After years I call her up out of the blue and say, hey you're a friend; want to be in my wedding? If she never speaks to me again, I wouldn't blame her," by now she was crying in her Mother's arms.

"Now…now…" her mother said, "Tiffany I'm not going to lie to you. What you did was pretty rotten and just plain wrong, but the love is there I can see it in you and I am sure she loves you still. That sort of love just doesn't go away. We just need to see if the rest fits into place; to tell you the truth, I don't think she would have agreed to come if she didn't still love you." With that her mother kissed her head and told her it was time to get up and get on with the day, then she walked out of the room.

Tiffany knew it was time to get up and she would in five more minutes she told herself, "OK, maybe ten..." with that she shut her eyes and went back to sleep.

...................................................................

Susan was trying to keep the fire going, but she wasn't having much luck at it when she heard the vehicle coming up the drive. As she hurried to the door, she saw the Jeep climb over the last snow bank before stopping at the front door.

"Come on," Steph yelled. "Get your coat, we're going to the Springs."

Susan wondered if Stephanie was going to be too hurt or mad and not speak to her on the ride. She was relieved that Stephanie was anything but quiet, she was cheery and talkative and Susan liked that in her. Many women she had known would have just sulked; she loved that Steph was different. She found it refreshing that she was very different on so many levels.

She had only known her for a few short days now and was impressed thus far. She also wondered if Steph knew what sort of an impact she was having on her thoughts? Stephanie spent a lot of time pointing out and talking about the area as they drove, more to keep Susan's mind off the drive, as the roads were very icy. At one point they hit a patch of black ice, and the Jeep did a complete donut before Stephanie could get it under control. Susan's heart was in her throat and pounding so hard she could not catch her breath, seeing how upset she was Stephanie pulled over and tried to calm her down.

"I know this has got to be hard for you," Stephanie said, with your accident the other day and all.

After calming her down, Stephanie put the Jeep back in gear. She was about to drive back onto the road when Susan reached over and took hold of her hand. "Wait, please," Susan said. She didn't know why she did it, but she spent the next hour sitting in the Jeep, on the edge of a snowy mountain road, telling Stephanie about her past. At least part of it, she told her all about the accident with Brittany, over eight years ago now, and how it was her fear still to this day when she rode with anyone.

"As long as I am the one behind the wheel in control I'm ok, but when I ride with anyone my stomach is in my chest the whole trip. It is as if I am holding my breath, and you know this is the first time I have ever told anyone about my fear."

"I am honored you trusted me enough to tell me, I totally understand. When my parents were killed on this very mountain I could not for the longest time even come back up here. Even now I get the Hebe jebes when I drive on it at times. I know they are watching out for me and that is what helps me through it."

It was at that point she realized she was still holding Steph's hand, and she felt very at ease about it. She also realized that the whole time she was telling the story, not once did Stephanie cut in, interrupt her, or look out the window as if she was bored. She sat and listened like she really wanted to know. Susan knew at that minute just what she had been missing these last few years.

"I guess we should get back on the road," Susan said. "I don't want you driving back in the dark, I want you to know, I have not felt so at ease about someone else driving, or just being with someone in a long time, thank you for listening to me rant and rave."

The rest of the drive was uneventful. Only when they pulled up in front of the house did Steph's heart sink a bit, as a beautiful woman she was assuming was Tiffany, ran out to greet Susan.

Susan seemed just as happy to see her also as she bolted out of the Jeep and into her arms. It was all Stephanie could do to keep a tear at bay.

It was several minutes before Susan seemed to remember Steph was still there. She said something to Tiffany and then walked over to the driver's side.

"Come here," Susan said as she grabbed Steph's hand pulling her out of the Jeep. After introductions were made she gave Steph a big hug. Stephanie tried not to let this feel like a final good bye when Susan said; "I want to thank you for all you have done for me and for just being there to listen." As she gave her a kiss on the cheek, Steph thought she saw a tear in the corner of Susan's eye.

"Drive safe," Susan said as Steph got in and shut the door.

"I will darling. I will also pull the car out and have it picked up so don't worry about it at all. You get this taken care of and remember I am here for you no matter what. You have my number; call me anytime, if you can get through."

As she waved, Stephanie thought she heard her said, "I'll see you in a few days." Or was it that she just hopped she had said that?

Stephanie cursed herself as she pulled out of the drive for looking in the mirror. She could no longer hold the tears back as she saw Tiff's arm go around Susan's waist.

Tiffany was eager to hear who had given her the ride and all about what happened over the last few days. She became frustrated when Susan was vague with her answers, and she let Susan know she was not happy about her attitude with the looks she gave and the exhaling often of her breath. Susan just pretended not to notice.

"How about us going to get something to eat?" Susan said. "I'm hungry. Let me call the rental place and let them know where their car is and arrange for another one, then I'll be ready to go."

"You won't need another one now that you're here," Tiffany said. "I have a couple of weeks off, that I was going to use for the honeymoon, so I can drive you around."

"No thanks, I think I would rather have a vehicle," Susan said. "I am not sure how long I will be here and well I just would rather be able to get around when I want. I would not want to put you out."

Sounding a bit hurt, Tiffany insisted it would be ok, but nonetheless Susan got on the phone and requested another vehicle. Tiffany heard her say this time she wanted the Jeep she was promised, with four wheel drive, and that she wanted it to be brought to her.

After she got off the phone she interrupted Tiffany's thoughts when she said, "ok, I'm ready to go."

During dinner they talked non-stop like old times, with ease. Susan had wondered if it would still be there, and she was relieved that it was.

"Do you know what ever happened to Michael?" Susan asked.

"Michael? I have not seen him since the day after the accident," Tiffany said. "When he came to the house that day, remember?"

Susan thought for a minute, "Isn't that when he saw us in our night things? Then turned red in the face and left without saying anything else?"

Giggling, Tiffany was remembering back, "You're right, it is," she said. "I have not even given him much thought;

what he must have thought seeing us like that," Tiffany said. "I just know he was thinking he was right all along about me being a lezbo," and with that both women giggled.

"How right he turned out to be," Tiffany thought. "Now if I can get a grip and just come to terms with it myself, I'll be doing good," she thought.

# CHAPTER 17

And this is how they spent the next several hours, sharing old stories. They both seemed to be staying away from any talk dealing with the here and now.

"You know what I want to do?" Tiffany said out of the blue. "I got myself a bee in my bonnet, and I want to go out to a club. How about it, are you game? I have not been dancing since you and I went to The Rainbow Club on the outskirts of campus, remember?"

"Dang girl, you need to get out more. That's been how many years ago now?" Susan said with a laugh, leading Tiffany to believe she was just a party animal.

"I say lets do it," Susan said. "Would you happen to know of any good clubs here in town, lesbian or gay ones?"

"Well, no," Tiffany admitted. "To be honest I don't know where any of that type of clubs are. I have heard there is one downtown called The Hide and seek off West Colorado Avenue but I have not been in that scene here in the Springs, so I don't know for sure. You would think as big a city this is that we would have some."

The next thing Tiffany knew, Susan flagged the waitress down and asked her if she knew of any lesbian clubs in town. This embarrassed Tiffany as she came here to eat all the time.

After the waitress went to find out from one of the other workers how to get to the club downtown, Tiffany went off on Susan. "What the hell are you doing? I come here to eat all the time, and I do not want these people looking at me funny or making comments about me behind my back. Please keep this stuff to yourself when you're with me," she added.

Susan was very annoyed, as well as taken aback at Tiff's reaction to an innocent question to the waitress; she could not believe that she was still denying it all even now. Not wanting to ruin the night, she just looked at Tiffany with anger and said nothing.

"Well then lets go find it ourselves," Susan finally said. As she stood up, she grabbed Tiff's hand to help her stand up. She was a bit shocked, as Tiffany quickly jerked her hand back.

Looking around quickly she wondered if anyone had just seen that along with her previous outburst. She then saw the look on Susan's face; Tiffany realized what had happened and tried to apologize.

"I guess I still have some of the old in me," she said in a nervous laugh. "I just don't care for public displays of affection."

Susan remained silent; she was steaming mad and knew to say anything would not be good right now.

They didn't have much trouble finding the club, once they made their way downtown.  Susan was the one that spotted the huge rainbow flag out front.

The place was packed, and after three shots of whiskey, Susan was feeling more relaxed. She wasn't much of a dancer, but she did like to watch others dance.  She was glad that the music now a day was so different that you didn't even need a partner; she spent a lot of time watching Tiffany dance.  Many other women in there were doing the same thing, Tiffany was very sexy and seemed to have all the moves, or maybe not. The way she looked when she moved, who would have noticed her missing a step or two?

The night was winding down and they both had had a good time. Tiffany dancing most of the night away never really coming around Susan at all, and Susan just relaxed watching the ladies dance. She even had fun shooting some pool.

The bartender called for last call and Susan feeling exhausted went to find Tiffany.

Tiffany was standing talking to some women out in the courtyard between clubs. The men's club was on one side of the courtyard and the women's was on the other. Susan thought it a nice set up; it made her feel comfortable.

"Hey babe," she said to Tiffany as she walked up behind her "you ready to head out, I'm beat?"

"Sure, I'll meet you outside in a minute," she said, and with that she turned her back on Susan and started talking to the others again.

As Susan sat in the car waiting on Tiffany, she realized she didn't know a lot about her any more. She didn't even understand her behavior. It had been years she reminded herself since she last saw her, and then laughed when she realized she had never understood her. It was only a couple more minutes when she came out to the car.

"Thank you," Tiffany said. "I needed this evening and I had a blast. I have not been out dancing for a long time."

"I enjoyed it also," Susan said dryly.

Nothing else was said until they pulled into the drive.

"Damn it," Susan said as they pulled into the drive.

"What is it?" Tiffany asked.

"Nothing, I am just mad that they didn't bring the Jeep this evening. If they don't bring it tomorrow, I am going to start getting pissed off."

Getting into the house proved to be a task in itself, as Tiffany had lost her house keys that evening somewhere. The only spare key was at her Mother's house, and it was almost three in the morning so neither wanted to wake her. They decided in their half drunk state that they could break in through one of the back windows without anyone calling the cops. The problem was they were laughing so hard their sides hurt and it was making it hard to climb in, being tipsy didn't help either.

"Hell, it only took us forty minutes to break into my own house," Tiffany said. "It's funny with you being the butch that you couldn't even climb through the damn window." With that statement, they both broke into new fits of laughter. After calming down a bit, Susan realized what time it was. "Dang girl, it is after 4:00 am and it has been a very long day for me, I think I will hit the bed. If you will be so kind as to show me where I am to sleep; I will bid you a fair night."

"Well," Tiffany slurred, taking Susan into her arms, "I was thinking that... well... maybe you could share the bed with me." She was stunned when she tried to kiss Susan and got no response from her at all.

Susan wasn't prepared for that statement or the attempted kiss. She knew if Tiffany had offered just three days ago, she would have jumped at it, but right now her head was still too mixed up.

"It's been a really long, tiring day and well, I think maybe..." Susan was trying to find the right words. "Tiffany, I don't mean to hurt you, but I would rather not."

Tiffany was hurt but didn't show it. "I see, well then let me show you to the guest room."

Susan lay there a few minutes thinking about the kiss. She was very perplexed because she had felt nothing. No electricity between them, no wanting, no nothing from Tiffany's kiss at all. It somehow was all gone. She was remembering Stephanie's soft warm kisses and how much she missed them.

It took Tiffany a bit to get to sleep also. She knew Susan had loved her. She pursued her, and now, she seemed to be the one aloof and cold.

"Maybe, she reasoned, it is just because I hurt her by asking her here to my wedding," she told herself. She still couldn't understand why Susan was being so cold to her. She had called the wedding off after all, and now she had the chance to be with her she thought. She had told Susan she loved her and wanted her back over the phone.

Damn... She said aloud She can't expect me to change over night I am at least trying, for some reason Tiffany thought she had did nothing wrong. "Maybe she did just have a really long day," with that as her last thought Tiffany rolled over and went to sleep.

Susan woke with a fright from a nightmare. She had been dreaming about losing Stephanie forever and being chained to Tiffany for eternity. Remembering what Freud had said about nightmares being the work of a guilty conscious she wondered what she had to feel guilty about. After a bit she rolled over and went back to sleep.

Tiffany woke up in a good mood and decided if she had to win Susan back she would do just that. She decided to wake her up with breakfast to get started on the right foot.

"Good morning sleepy head," Tiffany said, as she pushed the door open with her foot.

"What have you got there?" Susan asked, as she yawned and stretched.

"Breakfast," Tiff said with a smile. "I know you didn't eat a lot at dinner last night, so I thought I would bring you breakfast in bed."

"Wow, I'm impressed, to what do I owe this honor?"

"You have had a tough couple of days, and well, I wanted to do something nice, get a few brownie points maybe," Tiffany said as she giggled.

"It has been a rough few years," Susan thought, but just smiled at Tiffany.

She was cursing herself; all she could think about with this food in front of her was waking to the smell of Stephanie cooking for her. After only taking a few bites she thanked Tiff again, "Sorry, I am not too hungry. Let me get up and shower and dress, and we can get started with our day."

"Well I still need to shower also, we could save water," Tiffany said with a wink.

Seeing the look that came across Susan's face, Tiff quickly said, "I was just joking, and you can't blame a girl for trying can you?  Let's get going," Tiffany grabbed the breakfast tray, shaking her head on the way out the door.

Susan knew she was doing no one any good being here; she had to either leave or sit down and talk to Tiffany, and soon.

"Hey Tiffany, do you know anywhere we can go to get away and talk?" Susan asked as she came into the kitchen.

"Why do we need to get away? We can talk right here."

"I was thinking more on the line of somewhere outside, I feel like I have been cooped up. I am so use to being outside on the beach."

"Well, it's very nice out today and even warmer than yesterday. If you want to get out in the winter a bit, we can go to Palmer Park and sit up there and look at the city. I know there will not be another living soul up there this time of year," Tiffany said with a smile. "It should give us some alone time and we can talk."

"Great, lets do it. I am not big on snow as you know," Susan said "but maybe I can warm up to it, and the outside will do me some good to help clear my head I am sure."

"Let me get you some warm things to put on. I noticed you didn't really come prepared."

"I didn't have much with me and what warm things I do have, came from Stephanie. She let me borrow a few things."

"I see. Let me get you some better things then, these look like men's clothing," she said as she went to get some more things from another room.

# CHAPTER 18

During the ride they slipped a few times. Susan's knuckles were white from holding the armrest so tight. She spent most of the ride trying to figure out what she wanted to do for sure. She had spent so many years knowing only that she wanted to be with Tiffany, and that Tiffany didn't want her at all. Now something else had a major role to play in this little play of hers called life. Susan was no closer to an answer than when they started on their way to the park.

"They have a lot of the roads closed off up to the top of the park, but we can hike up if you want to." Tiffany said interrupting Susan thoughts.

"Sounds cold, but lets give it a shot," Susan said trying to be positive.

"Ok, hold on, let me grab my backpack" Tiffany said. "I have hot chocolate and lunch in here for us later."

As soon as Tiffany mentioned the hot chocolate, Susan's mind went right back to Stephanie. She couldn't keep from smiling to herself.

"What you smiling about?" Tiffany asked, catching Susan off guard.

"Nothing really," Susan offered, just thinking is all.

It wasn't a long hike up, but it took almost an hour. "Sorry I am just not very good in snow," Susan said, huffing and puffing. "I take two steps forward and slide back three,

I can't go on. I have got to rest for a minute, please, let's rest here."

"No, now come on," Tiffany said. "We're almost there, see the little clearing up there?"

Susan nodded her head that she saw it Tiffany said, "that's it...that's where we are going? Now come on you can make it," Tiffany said, laughing.

Tiffany took off. She was moving at a fast sprint when down she went, Susan burst out laughing,

"See, that's what you get for trying to show off," Susan joked.

"It's not funny," Tiffany whined. "I think I hurt my foot, I may have even broke it. Come help me up."

Susan stopped laughing and hurried to help her as fast as she could go, on the snow anyway. As she got to her, three falls later herself, Tiffany had her head down on her knees, making crying whining sounds. Susan bent over to see if she was all right just as Tiffany grabbed Susan's leg and pulled her down right on top of her.

"Psyc," Tiffany yelled, laughing as hard as she could. Susan slapped her arm as she tried to pill herself off Tiffany and get back to her feet, not having much luck.

"You big meanie," Susan said laughing also, "I was really worried about you."

They found getting up was much harder than getting down. As they got to the clearing, Susan saw the closed for the winter signs and got a bit worried. Tiffany saw what

Susan was looking at and smiled, "No worries love, that is so the city won't be sued if someone gets up here acting a fool and gets hurt."

For the first time since Susan got here she felt good about being here, thinking it was nice to hear Tiffany say love. It felt a little like old times.

It didn't take them long to cross the clearing to the knee-high wall, that surrounded the top of the little bluff, over looking the city. Tiffany got the little thermal blanket out that she had brought in the backpack for them to sit on. When they were both sitting looking out over the quite snowy city Susan began.

"Tiffany please don't say anything until I get done, if I don't get this all out I may not be able to at all, OK?"

"OK," Tiff promised.

"Let me start off by saying I am so sorry. I have had a bad attitude since I got here and I am truly sorry. It isn't you. I have had a bad attitude for several years really and well, ok; I guess it is you a bit, you and I. You did not do anything to me that I didn't let you do, and I realize this. Several years ago you left just like that, I had no answer at all, and I was and am still so confused about it all. All I felt when you got in your car and drove off was hurt, angry, confused, even betrayed in a lot of ways. Then, out of the blue, a few years later I get a call from you. I get on a plane, reluctantly mind you, to come to your wedding. I should have used those years to pull me back together but I didn't, and, I also..." Susan paused for a minute; "I also met someone else when I knew all hope for you and I was gone. Now after all this time you up and tell me you want me back, that we have a chance. I am even more mixed up than before. I have spent a long time loving you and wanting you, even when you no longer wanted me. What makes it worse is, I met someone else that I think I can really care about. I try to let go of you enough to give her a chance, but you're still right there haunting my waking as well as sleeping hours."

She could see what she was saying to Tiffany was hurting her, but she had to get it all out.

"I didn't tell you this to hurt you, and I'm sorry that it is. I don't think we can ever be anything unless we talk about this and to do so means to be honest. And in doing so...."

"Susan let me ask you something," Tiffany interrupted, "I know I promised not to talk until you were done, but I can't just sit and not say anything. I'm sorry but let me ask you some questions."

Susan just sat there looking at Tiff thinking back to how great Stephanie was to just listen without interrogating or interrupting or trying to fix everything that Susan was saying, she then said, "Ok, Tiffany, if you must, then go on."

"First, do you love me?"

"Tiffany, I cannot believe you asked me that. Hell yes I loved you when we lived together, I loved you when I first met you, and I have loved you from afar all these years, and yes I believe I still love you in some way. I am not sure if I am still in love with you though. I think some of that died when you phoned me about your wedding. Maybe even when you left me with that damn ditto. But I still did all of this. I didn't want to get on the plane; I didn't want to come here but I had to. I cannot say no to you even still."

"Ok then, second, how long have you had this other person and why would she let you get on the plane and come across country to be here with me?"

"Tiffany...the other person is...she is Stephanie, you met her when she dropped me off."

"I don't understand," Tiffany said. "I thought you just met her when you wrecked a few days ago."

Susan knew that she didn't need to answer Tiffany's question because the look in Tiffany eyes said it all; she now understood everything perfectly.

"So let me get this straight, this other person is Stephanie, You just met her and she is what is making you all confused about us? She is what is causing you to question your love for me?" Susan could tell that Tiffany was getting pissed off now, and her voice was growing louder. "You have been cold to me because of someone you just met? If you loved me, then why would she be an issue at all?" By now Tiffany was so mad she was crying.

It did Susan no good to try to explain anything, so she just sat while Tiffany had her fit. She felt surprised at herself. She thought she would feel some compassion

113

seeing her sitting there, crying, but she didn't. Something else struck her about what Tiffany had just said. Tiffany was right, if she still loved her then why would Stephanie be an issue at all. No one else had been an issue for all those years so why her now?

"So you have nothing at all to say about anything?" Tiffany finally said.

"Tiffany, I have said that same thing to myself for years."

"What are you talking about now?" Tiff asked. "You seem to be only saying negative things about me anyway, so go ahead and stab me some more."

"I am sorry you feel that way and what I was saying is…I have told myself many times that if she loves me how could she have left the way she did? If she loves me, how could she not let me go with her? If she loves me how can she be with a man or anyone else and marry them. If she loved me why did she deny me to everyone? I have tried to see it from your point but I can't Tiffany. I can't see it from any point other than my hurt. I do love you in some ways; this is the only thing I know. I am not sure if I even still like you as a person any more but I know part of me still wants you. That is what I am here to find out, if enough of me still wants us. I made a promise you will not like but nonetheless I made it, and I will keep it," Susan said.

"Do I even want to know what it is?" Tiff snapped.

Ignoring what Tiffany said Susan went on, "I promised Stephanie that no matter what the outcome with you and I, that I would go back and tell her in person".

"Oh I see," Tiffany said with a lot of attitude thrown in. "So if you DECIDED you want me I will just have to stand back and watch you go off to see her, I will have no say in it at all, and if it is her you pick..." she then let that thought trail off. "You know this is bull shit," Tiffany said. "You don't even know her, you met her and a few days later you're here with me. If it is she you wanted then why come here at all?"

"Tiffany, I came here to see you because I could not stay away. There was never any closure even back then and I think that we..."

Just as Susan was about to finish Tiffany broke in again. "You know what? I'm starving, lets eat and if you think we must, we can talk about this some more later, ok? I do not want to stand up here and talk about closure with you. We are both hurt and mad and will say things we are sorry for, so lets do this later."

"Yeah, ok Tiffany, whatever you want," Susan said trying to hide the indifference in her voice. She knew Tiffany had brought food with them but she nothing about it.

"Ok... then lets go, I'm getting cold and hungry out here anyway," Tiffany said.

# CHAPTER 19

She knew that Tiffany wasn't that hungry. This was just her way of avoiding the whole thing for as long as she could as she always did, and it angered Susan. However, she said nothing as they made their way back down the snow-covered hill.

Dinner was pretty quiet, neither one talked much even though they both had so much to say. Susan knew that the problem was that they were both stubborn, and neither one wanted to give in. Tiffany wasn't interested in hearing any more of what Susan had to say as it all seemed to be negative. She was used to getting her way all her life, and she didn't like the fact that this time was different.

"Tiffany?" Susan began.

"No," Tiffany said putting her hand up. "Not now. I can't Susan, I just can't talk about it any more right now."

"When then?" Susan asked. "We need to discuss this; it isn't just going to go away because you don't want to talk about it. I came here so we could talk about it together and decide together. Now can we please talk this through?"

Tiffany just shook her head no. She knew she had to talk about it sooner or later, but she just didn't want to face the fact that she may have made such a mess of things, that it was now too late for them. This isn't how she had planned for things to go.

Susan decided to let the subject drop. She didn't know what else to do.

As they were driving up the drive, Tiffany caught site of the Jeep sitting in the driveway. "Damn it, they brought it," she thought.

"Well, finally." Susan said, relieved. "I thought I was going to need to go there and get it myself."

Tiffany got out without a word and slammed the door, going into the house leaving Susan sitting there. After a few minutes Susan went into the house. She walked through the door and saw Tiffany sitting on the floor crying.

"I've lost you haven't I Susan?" Tiffany cried.

"Tiffany, I do love you. I always have, that's why I am here," she said as she walked over and took Tiffany into her arms. "Please baby, don't cry."

Tiffany, feeling a glimmer of hope, sat up wiping her eyes, "I don't mean to be a baby," she gulped.

Susan smiled at her, "You are not a baby; you're just hurting. Lets talk, ok?" She was trying to forget her own hurt and think of here and now.

"Ok," Tiffany said.

As they both sat there quiet for a few minutes Susan finally said, "I am all ready to talk and I don't even know where to start."

"Then I will start," Tiffany offered.

"When you and I first met I didn't like you and for a long time after I still didn't. I thought you were after Brittany.

117

Then one day I woke up and knew that I was right, I didn't like you, and I loved you. I truly thought I loved you only because of what had happened to Brittany. Never once did I let myself believe it was for any other reason because to do so would have been to admit I was gay. I chalked it up to her death and to it being the college thing to do, but it wasn't. I know that now. It's true that I could have never accepted or expressed it beyond our home. I could not even let our friends know. I was so ashamed, not of you; I was ashamed of us, but mostly of me. You were never anything but loving and kind to me, and look how I treated you. Then I ran, I ran as fast as I could go. Do you know I didn't even cry when I drove away and left you standing there that day, not one tear. I told myself all the way to Colorado that this must be the right thing to do; I am not even upset about it. It never even occurred to me that I was numb from shock."

After Tiffany grew quiet Susan said, "May I ask you something?"

"Please do," Tiffany said.

"When did you realize it Tiffany, when did you realize that you were in shock and that you loved, missed, and wanted me back? Was it after one year or after two years or even several years and why now? Was it that you were just looking for a way out of the wedding? Just what was it?"

Tiffany sat there for a minute before she answered.

"Susan, to tell you the truth, not until the other morning after my mother and I talked did I dare let myself think of it. I was sitting on this rock that I have over the years, made my own little place to go and think and be alone. I was sitting there thinking a few days ago after mother and I had our first real talk about all this, and it hit me then. I loved and missed you. My family would understand, I didn't think I had done anything wrong really; I just thought it took me longer to find myself. I guess I just sort of was hoping that you still loved me and wanted me. Then when I was on the phone the other night trying to get a hold of Larry, I realized that I loved Larry like a brother, nothing more. But what you and I had was passion, true passion. Giggles and butterflies even, you felt it didn't you? Well, didn't you?"

"Yes," Susan whispered. "I did feel that way from the beginning with you."

"So did I. I just didn't know it at the time," Tiffany said.

"The day Michael came to the house after the accident I was so scared he was going to tell everyone that he had seen you and I together. I think from that day on I was always listening with one ear at least, to hear if anyone was making fun of me behind my back. To tell you the truth, that night was the first night I knew who was in my dreams, it was you. I thought if we could just be together and no one knew it would be OK. It is no excuse, but I never had the chance to get use to being gay. I told myself I was just lonely, not gay, and after the fun of college real life would begin. I hear myself talk now and I know how bad I must have hurt you. I just want to make it up to you; I am so

119

sorry. Please give me one more chance; I promise it will be different."

Tiffany was uneasy as she talked because Susan was looking at her hard. Somehow Susan knew that Tiffany did believe it would be all right.

"Say something," Tiffany begged.

"You said you have your special place to go sit and be alone and think, when you did that over these years just how many times was it me you were thinking of?"

"Never," Tiffany whispered. "I just couldn't. That was all in the past, it wasn't real."

"It was always real to me Tiffany, always. My love for you, my wanting a life for us, all of it was real from the start. I was even willing to move back to a city that I despised just to be with you because it was where you wanted to be. To hear you say it has only been real for you for a few days now hurts more than anything you have said or done thus far to me. Would you feel OK about holding hands in public? Would you be ok with your friends and co-workers now knowing?"

"Yes I do believe I will be ok with all that," Tiffany said then added, "in time at least."

Seeing the look on Susan's face Tiffany went on to add, "These things take time Susan. You cannot expect me to change over night; you have been gay all your life. You have had time to get use to it, I haven't."

"No Tiffany, you're wrong. These things are natural when two people are in love. There is no getting use to how someone is. The very meaning of love is not being ashamed, or needing to change yourself for someone. I love you Tiffany the way you are, I always have. I came here to talk to you and try and find an answer. I can't because the more you say the more hurt and angry I get and as you said yourself nothing can be worked out like that. I don't know that I can trust your love anymore Tiffany or even my love for you. I think it is like a game with you, you feel like now that you have mommy's permission to love me that it is ok, so you can to come out and play. This is no game to me; I need time to process all this. I'm going to leave now at least for a few days, I need to see Stephanie. I promised her I would be back, and to tell you the truth I think she may hold more of my answers than you do. I'm sorry I don't have an answer but..."

"Let me guess," Tiffany interrupted bitterly. "You're going to go to her, oh I forgot, you got to keep the promise."

"I WANT to keep it," Susan said.

Seeing the tears in Tiffany's eyes Susan added, "This isn't goodbye Tiffany."

"Then what is it Susan? You say you love me, but how do you love me?" Tiffany asked.

"In these last few years I thought no one could replace the love I had for you Tiffany. Meeting Stephanie and trying to move on with my life, as I thought you had done, I found a part of me I had hidden away for so long. I have not lived at all in several years. For those few days on the mountain with her I started living again, I came out of my shell for the first time in years and I liked it."

"Answer me," Tiff yelled. "Damn you, answer me. How do you love me?"

"I don't know how I love you now," was all Susan could say. "I just don't know," as she got up to walk out of the room.

"Do you love her?" she heard Tiffany say. "Susan, do you love her?"

Without turning around Susan said, "YES, I do love her."

"Then I am done with all this," Tiffany yelled, "fuck you and the horse you road in on. You got the closure you have wanted Susan, the closure you came here for. Go to your new bitch, and please stay for more than a few days as it's over for me do not come back again. It is all in the past for me now."

"Stop this, you're just being mean and hurtful because you're hurt, and I am sorry for that. I didn't mean to hurt you, I've got to go," Susan said as she ran out of the house with tears she didn't know where was coming from.

# CHAPTER 20

It now seemed so long ago when Stephanie had dropped Susan off at Tiffany's house. She knew it had only been a couple of days but time seemed to stand still with her gone. The fact that Susan hadn't called her at all told Stephanie that all was working out with them two. She was trying not to give up hope, but felt it slipping away. Who was she kidding anyway? They had years together, and she had only a few short days with Susan.

She tried to keep herself busy so she wouldn't think about it. She spent the whole next day after dropping Susan off pulling Susan's car out of the embankment, like she had promised her she would. She also knew that the rental company would come for it, and on the off chance Susan came with them, she wanted it to be at her house and not on the side of the road. Steph knew at least she would get to see Susan again if only for a few minutes. Even though Susan said she would come back no matter what, she knew Tiffany would be foolish if she let her come back at all. All her hope was fading with each passing hour.

Stephanie was going stir crazy in the house with her thoughts of Susan, she hadn't heard from her in a couple of days now. She had all ready cleaned the house up several times, so she decided to make some hot cocoa and go around to Miss Rose's house. She had promised Miss

Rose she would come and get in some wood for her before the next storm set in, and she knew she could talk to Miss Rose about Susan, she would understand. Steph was always able to go to her and cry on her shoulder; they could just talk about anything and everything at all.

Miss Rose was a nice older lady whom Steph had known all her life. When Stephanie was very young they moved to this mountain and it was then that she met Miss Rose before her parents died. Miss Rose was always a recluse, she lived right around the bend from them, and she always seemed to be there for Steph when she felt no one else was. She never married or had kids, and Stephanie was thankful that she was still around; she was Steph's comfort blanket through everything.

When she wrote her first book it was Miss Rose that encouraged her to get it published, she had confidence in Stephanie when she didn't have any in herself. She knew if it had not been for Miss Rose she may have never even developed her writing skills, and then where would she be, she wondered.

It was Miss Rose that first talked to Steph about the birds and the birds so to speak. She had told Stephanie that the bees were the boys and that since Steph always had crushes only on the other girls around town that the bees had no place in their talks about love or matters of the heart. Miss Rose always made Steph laugh, and it never occurred to her to hide the fact that she liked girls, and not boys, when she was around Miss Rose. Her parents were always supportive of her no matter what, but they were sure it was a "PHASE" she would grow out of in time. Miss Rose knew it was just a part of who Steph was and not a phase at all and told her so. Yes, Steph felt like she was very lucky to have Miss Rose.

For years after her parents had died in a car accident on the snow-covered mountain late one night, Stephanie had refused to even come back. It was Miss Rose that made the drive to Kansas, where Stephanie was living after college, to convince her to at least come back for a visit, and to not blame the mountains. Miss Rose knew all it would take was for Steph to come back once and of course she was right. After the one visit Steph started coming at least once or twice a year. She said it was to get away to write, but Miss Rose knew it was more. She knew it was mostly to get away from whatever girl Steph had fallen for, to mend her broken heart and also to be there to help Rose out.

She loved Steph to death and she knew if she had a child of her own she could love it no more then she loved her, but she worried so about her. She knew her time was limited and she wanted Steph to find someone she could settle down with before her life was over, she didn't want to leave her alone in this world. She wanted it to be someone she could commit to. Miss Rose knew that Stephanie was so afraid of getting close to someone; she was afraid they too would be taken away from her as her parents were. She knew she got attached quickly but that it never lasted. She knew the right woman would come along for Stephanie if she had no all ready showed up. Miss Rose believed in fate and she believed fate brought Susan there for a reason.

Darkness had set in when Steph filled the thermos with hot cocoa and headed out to Miss Rose's place around 10:00 pm. "Dang it, I cannot believe I just hit the lock and me without my keys. Oh well, I'll break in later," Steph thought, telling herself she was not going to spend another night worrying over Susan. "What will be will be, easy words to say, harder to do," she thought. She knew she always fell easy for women but this felt different to her. Somehow she felt it was real this time and she even felt it could last. It was if what she had been searching for was now within her grasp, and yet she couldn't touch it yet.

It was such a clear night that she decided to walk to Miss Rose's house. She was just rounding the bend at Rose's when she thought she heard a vehicle climbing up the steep mountain road; she could hear the snow crackling and popping under the tires.

"Hello dear," Steph called out as she rounded the bend forgetting about the vehicle. She could see Miss Rose leaning against the shed, sitting on the woodpile. "What are you sitting out here in the cold for woman? You better get inside before you freeze to death. Rose?" Stephanie called out again as she waved her hand when she didn't answer, "I brought hot cocoa."

At that moment Stephanie knew something wasn't right. She dropped the thermos and ran to Miss Rose. When she got to her she could see Rose was bluish and cold as ice.

"OH MY GOD!" Stephanie cried. "No Rose, not you, wake up, please wake up." She knew she had to get her in the house; she could not let her stay out there any longer. It took all the strength she had to get Rose in. After laying her down on the floor she ran to the phone and grabbed it off its cradle. "Damn it, NO!" Stephanie cried. "It was dead."

She went back to Rose and held her head in her lap. She knew Rose was gone and could do nothing about it. "Why Rose?" she cried. "Why? I was going to get the wood in for you tomorrow. Damn it, why did I wait? Why didn't I come and do it today?"

Stephanie fell asleep with Rose's head in her lap, she awoke the next morning to the ringing of the phone. As she looked around, the night before came rushing back to her. Stephanie got up and went to the phone.

"Hello," she whispered into the phone.

"Rose, is that you honey, it's Lilly. Joe says the lines are only going to be up for a bit and that there going to go down again as bad as this storm is getting outside all ready, so I wanted to check on you while I could."

"No," Steph said, "This isn't Rose." She broke down and cried, "Miss Rose is gone and it's my fault. Please Lilly, send Sheriff Knox as soon as you can," and with that Stephanie hung up the phone. She knew Lilly, who ran the post office right next to the jail, would find him.

The storm that had moved in over night was looking pretty bad with each passing hour. It seemed like hours before the sheriff got there. He brought the coroner with him. They found Stephanie still on the floor holding Rose.

"Come on honey, I am sorry it took me so long to get here; The storm is getting pretty bad out there it is really coming down now." the sheriff said. "Come outside Stephanie, the coroner needs to get in here to her, we can't do anything for her now, she's gone."

"I tried to call last night when I found her but the lines were down, she was gone already," Stephanie said with fresh tears.

"The line only came back up a couple hours ago, you know how they go in and out honey. It isn't your fault Stephanie, you've got to know that, and Miss Rose was an old woman."

Steph learned later that Rose had died from old age and nothing more. They said it looked as if Miss Rose had been outside for at least twelve hours when Stephanie found her. They told her that she had died while outside, not from being outside. Still, Stephanie was sad that she had died alone. Knowing Miss Rose had no family, Steph took it upon herself to make all the arrangements, and all thoughts of Susan and anything else went out of her head.

........................................................................
..........

Susan didn't stop; she drove straight to Stephanie's house. She had to see her, things could not have gone worse at Tiffany's. It was slow going as she still didn't have the hang of driving on this stuff, and everything kept running through her head. Tiffany and Stephanie and the past and the now, she was so lost. Was what she had with Tiffany (which she now knew was only one sided all along) real and still there enough, she doubted it and was what she had started to feel with Stephanie real and not just rebound and enough to last? She kept asking herself how could it be rebound? It had been several years after all.

It was close to 10:00 pm, well past dark when she passed the accident site. There were no lights except for the full moon reflecting off the snow on the mountain, yet she could see that the car was gone.

"Good, they came and got it already," she thought, but as she rounded the hill to Steph's drive a while later she saw it sitting in the driveway. It looked so out of place to her sitting where the tractor had sat just a few days before. She could tell Stephanie had struggled to pull it up here because she hand not bothered to remove the chains yet, and it was still hooked to the tractor sitting in front of it.

Susan sat in the Jeep for a few minutes not knowing what to do. There were no lights on in the house and as it was only 10:25 pm she didn't expect Stephanie to be in bed already. Deciding she could not wait in the Jeep all night, she figured Stephanie would not get to mad being woken up this once Susan thought with a smile.

# CHAPTER 21

A chill ran through Susan as she got out of the Jeep. She didn't think she would ever get use to this sort of weather; she hated it as a kid. She knew she would not grow to love it now, but she figured if nothing else she could grow to accept it. She slipped and slid all the way to the front porch. As she stepped on the bottom step her left leg went right out from under her and down she went. She was laughing as she tried to get up, grabbing the rail to help herself up.

Once on the porch she thought she heard something. It was faint but she could have sworn she heard Stephanie cry out. She listened real close but heard nothing else other than the wind whipping the snow and ice everywhere. She knocked on the door. Hearing nothing, she knocked again.

She decided to go on in and wake her up. As she turned the door handle she was surprised to find that it was locked. "Damn it," she said, "she's left already." Steph had told her that the only time she ever bothered to lock the door was when she closed the house up to go back to Kansas.

Susan was getting worried now and cursing herself that she had not even bothered to call Stephanie to make sure she was going to be here. "Damn it," Susan said to herself, "I'm such an idiot."

There was an old swing on the porch, so Susan sat down just about freezing her butt off as she did. However, she was too numb in her thoughts to notice how frozen the swing was. "It all meant nothing to Stephanie," Susan said aloud to no one. "I told her I would be back and she didn't even wait for me to get back here to give her the answers I came up with, she just left, just like that, as if I didn't mean anything to her. Hell, maybe we really didn't have anything after all, it was just only a few short days together."

Almost in tears Susan decided she would head back to the Springs. She didn't want to be stuck here in the Jeep overnight, "With the way my luck has been going," Susan thought, "I would probably freeze to death or something."

Getting out of the swing proved to be a hard task as she was stuck to the wood. As she pulled she heard a ripping sound that Susan knew wasn't good. Sure enough she felt a draft as she stood all the way up, she had to laugh at herself as she looked at half her backsides fabric stuck to the swing. "Only me," she thought, "only me."

About to pull out of the drive she caught sight of the rental car again with the tractor still attached to it and she didn't think that Stephanie would have left without making sure the rental people had picked up the car as she told her not to worry about it that she would have it taken care of. In the back of her mind she knew that Steph had not went back home to Kansas, thinking she may be at her friends or something but not knowing when she might be back, she decided that she could not just leave without leaving a note and her number in Florida, as she decided she was heading back home in the morning. So she pulled back up the drive. "Stephanie may never get it but at least I know I tried once more, or as they say on TV, I cared enough to leave the very best," she chimed to herself. "Ok, get a grip girl," she told herself, "you're just being silly now." As she wrote the simple note out it said.

(*Stephanie, you came into and touched my life when I had given up all hope of ever being able to let the past go. I need to thank you for that. Nothing was worked out with Tiffany; I do know now that she isn't whom I want to be with. I could not get you out of my head, and I had to come here to see you. I am so sorry I didn't call, as the lines were down a lot, I had so hoped we could talk and figure out what we both wanted. I am saddened I have missed you; I didn't think you would be going back to Kansas so soon if indeed this is where you have gone. I hope I didn't mess your swing up as I sort of got stuck to it. Sorry baby, if you do get this note here is my number at home, I will be leaving tomorrow morning to head back to Florida, if the weather holds up that is. If it doesn't then I have no clue as to what to do. Please call me at 813-555-7664)*

*(PS. I think I am in trouble with how I feel about you.)*

After dropping the note in the mail box so she didn't need to get out of the Jeep again with her bare backside she made the long drive back down the mountain, in tears most of the way. It was well after 4:00 a.m. when she got to

Tiff's. She wished she didn't have to face Tiffany at all, but she knew she had to get her things. She figured Tiffany would be mad since she told her not to come back, she was half thinking or hoping that Tiffany would have her things on the porch waiting for her. She knew she wanted to see her; she didn't want to leave things the way they had ended earlier. She had decided on the drive back that she had to get on with her life without Tiffany, not wanting to hurt her but knowing she had to go on. She loved Tiffany, but she now knew she wasn't in love with her.

Tiffany heard the Jeep pull into the drive; she had not been able to sleep at all. As she looked out the window she saw Susan getting out of the Jeep and fresh tears started streaming down her face, this time they were not the sad tears she had been crying all night. She knew it was Susan coming back and she was now crying tears of relief because she thought her mouth had ran Susan off for good this time.

As Susan was about to ring the bell the door swung open and Tiffany rushed out and took Susan into her arms.

"Oh baby, I am so glad you decided to come back to me, I was so scared you would just stay there with her after what all I said," she added in a snide tone.

"I left my clothing here Tiffany, and you should know me better than that. I would have at least came back to say good-bye and well to tell you the truth that is one of the reasons I did come back. I have decided that I am flying home in the morning."

Tiffany let Susan go and just looked at her.

"Why?" Tiffany pleaded. "Was it because of what I said? Was it because of the mean things I said to you?"

"Tiffany, try to understand, please. At first I thought I should not have come here at all but I am glad I did, we needed closure. I love you and will always treasure what we had. It has been too long Tiffany and too much has happened. Seeing Tiffany about to say something Susan went on, "and before you say it, Stephanie had nothing to do with this decision of mine, she wasn't even home. I have spent the whole day and night thinking about it as I drove. This is the only thing that feels right. I have put you on a pedestal for years and that is my fault, I should never have done that because no one could live up to that. It was my fault for doing it. It was just a way for me to go on living without needing to live. It was safe if I had you even just in my heart then I didn't need to feel anything anymore. I hope you find yourself, or what you're looking for, but I just can't be that one anymore."

"Why can't you look at me Susan when you say that?" Tiffany asked through her tears.

"Because I know I am hurting you and I do not want to. I know if what you and I had were still there, I would not have fallen for Stephanie. You made me realize that when we were talking before. You said those same words to me, and that was when I knew you were right. Tiffany I did fall for her, And even though it now seems that she and I are not going to work out, it doesn't change the fact that you and I are no more, nor does it change the fact that you and I have not been for a long, long time. I will not use you like that, I am so sorry. I will leave first thing in the morning if you don't mind me spending the night here."

"No, of course I don't mind," Tiffany said with no emotions in her voice at all.

As Susan thanked her and turned to walk away Tiffany noticed the big hole in the back of the pants but said nothing. Susan decided to pack so she would be ready to go at first light, which was in less than three hours.

Tiffany knew nothing she could say would help as she watched Susan go. "What could she say?" she thought. "I don't really blame her, but I do blame Stephanie."

Susan woke to Tiffany coming into the room singing, carrying the newspaper under her arm and some fresh coffee and bagels, Susan wondering what was going on with the mood change as Tiffany sat the platter down and went to open the curtains wide.

# CHAPTER 22

"Morning sleepyhead," Tiffany said as chipper as if last night had never happened at all.

"Morning Tiffany," Susan said in surprise. "You're very upbeat this morning, did I miss something?"

"Well, Tiffany started. "I hope you're not too mad and I promise I didn't make a pack with God or the devil to do this," she added with a smile, "but I don't think you're going any where today, it is coming down in buckets outside and the weather girl says it will be this way the rest of the day, maybe even longer."

Susan threw the covers back going to the window, "No, not this morning," Susan groaned. "I have a flight today, damn it, I hate snow." Looking out the window Susan could see nothing but snow everywhere; she saw that the Jeep was even half buried under a large snowdrift all ready.

"I just knew it," she said aloud.

"Knew what?" Tiffany wanted to know.

"Oh, I was just thinking aloud, I told myself last night with the way my luck was going I would have froze to death if I tried to sleep in the Jeep instead of making the long drive back here, and see, just look out there, I would have."

"Come on Susan, let's just make the most of this. Maybe this is the work of a higher power trying to tell us something," Tiffany offered.

"Tiffany I hope you understand what all was being said last night, but please lets just make the most out of this, ok? No pressures or anything, is it a deal?"

Tiffany thought for a minute and knowing it would be the best thing to do by making the most out of the bad situation, "sure," she said, a bit weary. "Ok, you're right, lets make the most out of it."

Thinking for a minute Susan added, "I never wanted to not be friends with you Tiffany, so what do you say, friends?"

"Friends at the very least if I have anything to do with it," she thought but all she told Susan was, "sure, great friends."

They decided to spend the day together outside. Susan was sure she had cabin fever and didn't want to stay in any longer. They both seemed to have a lot of fun outside, less pressure to talk Susan thought.

"Wow, for someone that doesn't like the snow you sure seemed to be adjusting well to it," Tiffany commented.

"Well we did say we were going to make the best out of the situation now didn't we?" Susan said with a smile.

"Good girl," Tiffany thought. "Good girl."

Over tea that night Tiffany was lost in her thoughts that all was working out better than if she had wished for the snow and Susan in her thoughts wondering where Stephanie had gone off to and if she had gotten back and found her note.

"I think I will turn in early," Susan said, still lost in her thoughts of Stephanie. She wasn't feeling well, she seemed to be getting light headed more and more and didn't know why. "I'll see you in the morning." With that she went upstairs and went to bed, leaving Tiffany sitting there alone.

..............................................................................
............

It was well past noon when Sheriff Knox and the coroner took Rose's body away. Feeling drained, Stephanie went home to make arrangements and to shower. As she got to her front door she remembered she had hit the lock by mistake the night before, so she knew the only way in without breaking a window was to climb on the swing and go through the little crawl space above it.

As she brushed the snow off so she could get a good footing she noticed the material stuck to the swing, she tried to pull it off but it wouldn't budge. Perplexed as to how it got there she decided to worry about it later, she knew it had not been there yesterday morning because she had sat on the swing after one of her cleaning spells. All she could think of right now though was the shower.

When that was done all she wanted to do was sleep. Hours later she woke with a start and for a minute she thought it had all been a dream but then she knew it wasn't. Rose was really gone and Steph's sadness overwhelmed her again.

After putting the kettle on to make some coffee Stephanie went to start a fire to try and get some of the chill out of the air. She didn't know how long she sat there looking into the flames when she heard the kettle whistling at her. After her coffee she knew she had to go out and get some more wood in, knowing she didn't have enough to last through the night let alone throughout the storm. She had slept most of the day away it would be dark pretty soon.

As Stephanie rounded the side of the house on her way out to the woodshed, she noticed her mailbox door opened a bit. She knew it had not run today due to the weather, so she forgot about the wood and went to see what was up. As she opened the paper she found inside the box her hands shook as she read the words. "She did come back," Stephanie thought, "but when? Oh no it must have been last night when I found Rose."

Rereading the note she knew she had came last night, because of the swing. As she hurried into the house all she wanted to do was call Susan. She didn't know when Susan would be arriving home or if she could even fly out in this weather, she knew she came by some time last night so she should be home sometime today as the note said she would be going back this morning. Stephanie knew if she wasn't there she could at least leave a message so it would be the first thing she heard when she arrived home. "Damn it," Stephanie said out loud when she picked up the phone and it was dead again.

141

Stephanie decided all she could do was get some rest tonight as tomorrow was going to be a busy day with the funeral and all, if she could even get off the mountain to go to it. She had decided to not have a wake. Miss Rose didn't have family and most of her friends were too old to make it out to go anyway. Robert had called earlier before the lines went down when she was asleep, his message said that he needed to see her within the week and that if he could be of any help just let him know, but he being the town lawyer made Stephanie nervous. She knew to hear what he had to say just made it that much more final.

As she tossed and turned all night, a worry crept into her mind. "What if the storm set in before the plane took off? Would Susan be sitting at the airport, she said in the note that nothing had worked out with her and Tiffany, so would Tiffany let her stay there? Could she get a room if Tiff said no? And worse yet, if she said yes to let her stay there what could that mean?"

More perplexed than before she was now wide awake. "Well, at least its 5:00 am," she thought to herself as she got out of bed coming to a decision, she had made a plan she felt would work. Knowing now that after the funeral she was going to try and make it to the Springs to find Susan or at least get a hold of Tiffany and find out what she could. She was going to find Susan if it meant going to Florida herself, she felt a little better with a plan.

It took her all of thirty minutes to pack. She wasn't sure what she would do when she got to where ever Susan was, but she knew she didn't want to come back until she had at least talked to or saw Susan, she would do whatever it took to get Susan to want to be with her. Robert would just need to wait, she scratched out a note to him explaining that she needed to leave town for a few days and that she would call to set up a meeting with him as soon as she got back. She figured if she didn't have a chance to talk to him at the funeral to explain, she could at least give him the note.

# CHAPTER 23

"Guess what?" Tiffany said as Susan came down the stairs, "Mom is coming over today if she can get through. I heard on the radio that they are going to clear Academy Road this morning, if they get to it she will be able to get through. I know she is so excited to get to see you again."

"So the phone lines are up?" Susan said hopeful.

"No, afraid not." Tiffany said in her light tone. "We have a standing brunch date each week. I know she has wanted to see you, but she has been staying away to give us some time."

"Do you have any idea when the lines will be back up or when the airports will open back up?" Susan asked.

"Well, the radio said the one in Denver is open but we would play havoc getting there, as the roads are a mess, so I guess it is best just to wait it out here," she added.

The visit with Mable went well, it was hard for Susan to pretend like she was having a great visit. She hated not being honest, even if she was only half lying, but Tiffany said she didn't want to worry her mother. So to save peace Susan agreed to at least not bring anything up.

When brunch was over and Mable left, Susan decided she was going to go for a drive, as Mable didn't talk as if the roads were that bad. Susan even thought she caught an angry look on Tiff's face when her Mom had said that.

"OK sounds like a good idea, let me get my coat," Tiffany said.

"No, that's OK," Susan said, "I think I want to drive around alone."

"Oh no," Tiffany said. "You don't know how to drive in this stuff, and I would be too scared for you to be out alone in it."

Trying to brush it off to no big deal Susan smiled and said, "I'm a big girl, I'll be fine, and I've been driving in it for several days now. And besides I have a city map, so no need to worry."

As she grabbed Steph's jacket she had been wearing, she headed out the door. She knew Tiffany wasn't happy with her right now, but when she had decided to move on she decided to not let herself get involved with how Tiffany felt about any of it. She had decided to not pussyfoot around any longer to spare feelings. She was ready to live again she thought. She found that the roads were not that bad at all in some places.

.................................................................
......


"It was a lovely funeral dear," Lilly said To Stephanie as she hugged her. "Miss Rose was so proud of you dear, you know you brought her such joy to her life."

"Yes, I know," Stephanie said with tears in her eyes. "I miss her so very much all ready. At times I catch myself making a mental note to share something with her later when I see her, then it hits me that I won't ever see her again. My heart thinks it is all a dream, but it isn't a damn dream."

"I understand dear, it's to be expected," she said as she hugged Stephanie again, "you know she thought of you like her own daughter. She was so very fond of you."

"Thank you," Stephanie said.  "I think...thought the world of her also." Stephanie corrected with fresh tears that she was trying to gulp back.  "Please excuse me Lilly, I need to speak to Robert for a minute," as she made her way over to where he stood talking to Sheriff Knox.

"May I please speak with you Robert, sorry to interrupt sheriff," Stephanie said.

"Sure dear, let's go over here," he said. As he took her arm to help lead her across the room so they could talk in quiet.

"I need to go away for a few days, I am not sure when I will be back but would it be OK with you if I just make an appointment when I get back in town?" Stephanie asked.

"Well," he began with a worried look on his face. "How about if after the funeral is over you stop into my office and we talk then? This really can't wait that long. I hate to do this on a day like today but..."

"No, no that's fine," Steph said, a little relieved. "I was not planning on heading out until this afternoon anyway," she added.

"How about in forty-five minutes I meet you there, then?"

"That's about all the time I need Stephanie said, I need to make the rounds, you understand."

"Yes dear I do," Robert said, seeming wearier than Stephanie had remembered, maybe they all were a little older and wearier. "Forty-five minutes then."

It didn't take as long as they had thought it would, and thirty minutes later Stephanie was all ready waiting in his office.

"The service was pretty good don't you think?" he asked as he came in the door. "Well as far as that sort of thing goes anyway," he added

"Yes it was very nice," Stephanie said, and she meant it. She knew Miss Rose would have enjoyed it herself.

"Come on in while I hang my coat up hon; you can go ahead and start flipping through that file on my desk, do you see it? The blue one marked Miss Rose? This should not take too long we just have some things we need to go over and sign."

About fifty minutes later Stephanie emerged from Roberts's office in more of a daze than she was already.

..............................................................................
.........

It was only around 5:00 p.m. when Susan pulled into the airport parking lot, but it was already getting dark. Not knowing why she was there, even the guard at the gate said it was still closed to flights, she decided she just had to try and get some answers.

"Hello, May I help you?" the peppy girl behind the counter asked as Susan approached her.

The airport felt so weird to her, because other than a few workers and some passengers that were stuck here from laid over flights, the place was dead.

"I sure hope so," Susan answered. "I'm Susan Back, I had a reservation for a flight this morning that was cancelled because of the weather and I need to get home. I need to see if I could book another one ASAP?"

"Ok then let me have a look-see… Hum…" she said as she was typing away on the computer "these things are so slow in bad weather" she remarked patting the top of her screen, "ok I'm ready, so tell me first where are you heading?"

"I'm going to Key West in Florida," she added unsure if the girl would know where that was. "If you can even get me to Miami, I would be happy and I could then figure the rest out from there," Susan answered.

"I understand, anywhere other than this cold place, Ok lets see. Well if you can get to Denver we have one leaving tonight, but you would need to hurry to make it in time."

"How about from here, I do not want to drive all the way to Denver," Susan broke in, "I'm just not great driving on this stuff," she added.

"As of right now, tomorrow evening at the earliest is about the best I can do as long as this weather holds. You never know around here, but I could get you on the one tonight from Denver if you wish?"

"No thank you, the one tomorrow will be fine I guess," thinking to herself, "I can wait one more day." After handing her the credit card to book the flight for tomorrow evening, she thanked the girl.

"I think before I head back out in this snow I will get something to drink; would you please direct me to the lounge?" Susan asked. "I need to calm my nerves."

Stephanie spent most of the drive to the Spring's thinking of what Robert had said to her and how she was going to get Susan to come back. Miss Rose was still there for her even now, she could feel her in the Jeep that once was Rose's but now belonged to Stephanie. "Thank you Rose," she said to herself. It was almost dark when she got to the Springs, she was headed to Tiff's house to try and get some information out of her before it was too late.

As she pulled up in the drive she was praying Susan was there. Not seeing the rental Jeep she decided to go to the door, she was met at the door even before she knocked, by Tiffany.

"Hi," Stephanie said. "I don't know if you remember me or not, I am Stephanie. I was going to go straight to the airport to see if I could get any information on Susan, but I thought I would try here first. Would she by chance be here?"

"Nope!" Tiffany said. "And hell yes, I remember you all right," she added in her drunken tone.

"Could you please tell me where Susan is or how I might reach her?" Steph asked.

"Sorry, I can't give that kind of personal information out about my woman," Tiffany said in her bitchiest tone, as she shut the door in Steph's face.

Stephanie stood there stunned for a minute, "How dare her," she thought, then decided she would probably act the same way if she had just lost Susan. She was determined to not let Tiffany get to her, hurrying to the Jeep, knowing she had to get to the airport before it closed.

# CHAPTER 24

"Hello, May I help you?" the girl behind the counter asked.

"I sure hope so," Stephanie answered. "I do not have time to go into it all, but I need some information. Did you have any flights that leave today heading to the east coast? If so, may I please ask if a very important friend of mine was on there?"

"Well, all I can tell you is we didn't have any flights go out today due to the weather. I would not be able to give you the passenger list anyway; your friend may have taken one out of Denver though, as they have been running most all day."

"Damn it," Stephanie said, looking very distraught.

The girl feeling sorry for her offered, "Tell you what, leave your name, number and your friends information and I will post it up here next to the computer, in case she checks in here. On the off chance someone puts two and two together with her name she may at least get the note from you. We don't normally do that but I will this once."

Knowing she had no other choice, she wrote the information down for the girl. Stephanie thanked her and headed to the door, not knowing what to do from there.

"Excuse me, Miss…Stephanie," she said looking at the note, "excuse me."

Hearing her name, Stephanie turned back around.

"Could you please describe your friend for me?"

As Stephanie described Susan a smile came across the girl's face.

"Here," she said, as she handed the note back to Steph.

"What's wrong?" Stephanie asked.

"I think the person you are looking for may still be here, check in the lounge," the clerk said pointing to the escalator.

"No way," Stephanie said. "Are you for real?" not waiting on an answer, she hurried to the lounge.

"Susan!" Stephanie yelled, running up the escalator not caring who might hear or see her. Surprised at hearing her name, Susan looked up.

"Oh my God!" was all she could say as she just stared at Stephanie hurrying towards her. "What are you doing here? How did you know I was here?" Susan asked.

"It's a long, long story," Stephanie said, taking her into her arms, right in the middle of the lounge.

"I will tell you all about it later. Right now I just need to hold you baby; I was so scared and worried that I had lost you for good."

Stephanie didn't know, she couldn't know, how much Susan needed her there and how much she needed her to hug her even right there in public, especially right in public. She knew Stephanie wasn't ashamed of them at all, no matter who may be around or see and she hoped Tiffany one day found that sort of love also.

As they got to the parking lot, Susan remembered that they both had vehicles there.

"Hold on Steph, ok?" Susan turned around and ran into the building. After a few minutes she emerged with a smile on her face.

"What did you do?"

"I hope it is ok with you, and I am sorry I didn't ask, but I could not bare to be away from you. I called the rental company and told them where there Jeep was and to please pick it up. They were not too happy about it, but then when I reminded them about the escapade with the Escort, they seemed more than happy to come get it, "Not" but hey they will live, I don't want to be away from you. Is that ok?" Susan said soft and shyly.

"I just know you are not asking me if it is ok," Stephanie answered back. "Lets get your things out of the Jeep before I hurt you," she said with a giggle.

"I don't have anything in the Jeep except a map, I need to run to Tiffany's house real quick. All my things are there."

"Ohh!" Stephanie said.

"What is it?" Susan wanted to know. "Is something wrong?"

"Well," she started, "I do not think that it would be a good idea for me to go back over there."

"Why would you say that?" Susan wanted to know.

"I went by there before I came here, and well let's just say I received less than a warm welcome. She was a bit drunk, and she told me you were her woman so she could not give your personal information out to me. Then she shut the door in my face."

"I am so sorry honey. I don't want you to be put in the middle of all this mess. I want you to know I am not her woman and have not been for a long time. She never wanted me to be and now that I have found someone else that I do want to be with, guess what? She now has decided that she wants me. Well I have given it a lot of thought, and this time I am doing what I want to do, being with you is what I want. I will run over there alone and get my things so you don't have to be around her again," Susan said.

"Hell no, I do not want you to go alone, so Miss Tiffany will just need to get over herself," Stephanie said with a smile.

"Thank you," Susan said, giving her a hug.

"Honey, please do not ever be sorry, because if you weren't here, and I wasn't in the middle we would have never met. No sorrys, ok?"

Smiling, Susan agreed, "ok!"

"I have something to tell you Susan. Remember Miss Rose? The neighbor lady who's Jeep I have?"

"Yes I remember her," Susan said. "She is the one that loaned you the Jeep to bring me here the first time, right?"

"I am sorry to say," Stephanie said but "she died the other night."

"Oh no, I am so sorry Stephanie. I know you were very close to her."

"Thank you baby. I want to talk to you about some other things also, but first, lets get this taken care of, ok?" she added.

After filling Susan in about the rest of her visit to Tiff's, the ride was pretty quiet. Both women were lost in their own thoughts happy to be with one another.

# CHAPTER 25

"Hello, Tiffany are you there?" Larry called out. "I know it's late, but we need to talk."

"Hello," Tiffany said, as she opened the door. "I am sorry it took so long; I didn't know it was you until you called out. Come in please."

"You look awful Tiffany, are you sick? I can smell what's wrong, why are you drunk? Why were you not answering the phone or door? I have tried to call most of the evening," then seeing the look on her face and the tears in her eyes he said, "I'm sorry," Larry said, "I didn't mean to sound hateful. I was just getting worried about you, I still care for you, and I hope you know this." Somehow seeing her cry made his anger and hurt subside a bit.

"I care for you also, I always have" she said "it's nothing," Tiffany offered, not wanting to let him know what a mess Stephanie had made of things.

"Stop it right now," Larry said. "If nothing else we have always been able to talk about anything with one another, well most anything," he corrected, so talk to me. "I'll tell you what, go wash your face and blow your nose, and I will make some tea for us ok? Then we can talk."

"Well, now you look a little better. Come here," he said, "sit down and talk to me, tell me what is wrong. I have a feeling," Larry said lighthearted, "that all this hurt and crying and being upset isn't over the wedding not going as we had planned."

Tiffany had to smile a little bit on that one. "You always did know how to make me smile, didn't you? Can you ever forgive me? I thought what I felt for you was one thing and it turned out to be another. I do love you just not the way you deserve to be loved by a wife," Tiffany could barely get the words out between sobs. "I truly never knew I was a...a...see I can't even say the word yet," she started sobbing even harder now.

"What I don't understand," Larry said, "where is your friend, what is her name, Sara or Susan?"

"Her name is Susan," Tiffany sobbed.

"Why is she not here with you now, you need her here with you?"

It took Tiffany a long time to get the story out, and when Larry just sat there looking at her not saying anything; Tiffany grew nervous.

"Tiffany," Larry said after a long pause, "'I will be honest with you, but I will tell you now, I do not mean to hurt you. I know what I am about to say to you will hurt you, but it needs to be said. Please try to listen objectively I need to say this. You are being selfish and self involved and just plain mean. You are blaming another woman, whom you do not even know, for what all has happened or gone wrong in your life. First of all she had nothing to do with what all happened in college, that was all your doing. If Susan has fallen for this person now, it is because she had no one for years and she was trying to move on. When she thought you were getting married to me, she had no reason at all to think there were any hope for you two any more. Take yourself out of the picture and look at it. Here let me break it down to you as I heard you say. First, you fall in love with a woman and you are so ashamed of the fact that she is a woman, that you will not be seen with her at all. You will not let anyone know, you even go so far as to deny her to your family and friends, knowing she loves you enough to stay anyway. Then, when you're ready for the 'REAL' world as you put it, you say good-bye just like that, as if what you both had was nothing. Then, years later, you call her out of the blue to be in your wedding, not caring about her. She waited on you for years and then when she knew you had really moved on, she had to accept that. Circumstances gave her hope of also being able to move on, and it was hard on her not wanting to hurt you and all. She had made her mind up, and she did move on and now all you can do is sit here and feel sorry for yourself blaming some other woman for all your pain. You do not even know her. Before this night is over Tiffany, I want you to try and forget your pain for a minute and see what others are seeing and feeling, not just yourself, all other parties included. I am your friend, as I have been for a long time now and will continue to be, you may have been hiding from yourself but others saw, and you say you didn't know who you really were. I don't believe that for a minute. I believe you knew all along in one way or the other, and drinking yourself silly will do nothing to help anyone."

"How do you mean others know things?" she asked.

"Think about it, is all I can say. I am going to go now and give you some time to think." Giving her a big hug, he then looked into her eyes and said, "honey, yes I forgive you," with that he was gone.

..................................................................................
............

After riding in silence for a bit, Susan turned to Stephanie, "You know, after the last few days we have had I think it better to just hold off on getting my things for a few days, that is if you don't mind me wearing more of yours," Susan said with a smile.

"Of course I don't mind, but are you ok with that? I don't mind going over with you."

"I know and it isn't that, I just do not feel like being there right now. You and I have a lot to talk about; let's just use this time for us, ok? Anyway, it's just clothing and my toothbrush, I can get them anytime or never even." she added.

Stephanie didn't like the last part, "Susan, if you don't go get them, or at least face Tiffany, we will always have that left unresolved. I do not really want anything hanging over our head."

"I will get them, I mean, we will take care of it at a later date, just not tonight. Lets have a few days for us, OK?"

"That's fine by me, I'd like you all to myself anyway tonight," Steph said with a twinkle in her eyes.

"I have four more days before I told my house-sitter Mr. Edward I would be back. I was just trying to head back today because I thought you were gone, and I didn't think I had a reason to stay here anymore."

"Why would you think I was gone?" Stephanie asked a bit perplexed.

"Well, I am embarrassed to say this, but when I went to see you the other evening the lights were off and I thought I heard you cry out. After you didn't come to the door, I tried your handle and it was locked. And well you…"

"I remember," Stephanie broke in. "I told you I never ever lock the doors when I am staying there only when I close the house up to go back, since I felt so safe there. When you found it locked you thought I had left. I locked it on accident that night when I found Rose dead, what you heard was me crying out when I found her, but why ever would you be embarrassed to tell me that?" Stephanie asked.

"I didn't want you to think I tried to break into your house is all. So would you mind if I spent the rest of my time off with you?"

"Heck no," Stephanie said. "And I hope to convince you to stay a lot longer than just that, before it's over with," she added.

# CHAPTER 26

"The drive back was very slow going," Stephanie, thought Susan was asleep; she had laid her head on Steph's shoulder a while ago. Her breathing was slow and even, and she had not said anything for a long time.

"I wonder," she said into the dark night, making Stephanie jump almost out of her skin.

"Oh my, I thought you were asleep; you about scared me to death," Stephanie said placing her hand over her heart emphasizing the point.

"Sorry Stephanie. I didn't mean to scare you, I was just enjoying the ride and being close to you is all. I was also wondering how things went from where they were at a week ago to the way they are now. Do you believe in fate, or Karma as some call it?"

"Well to be honest, I don't believe I did, well not until you smashed the car into my mountain that is. Now I believe more and more each day," Stephanie said with a smile. "Why do you ask me that?"

"No reason really," Susan said with a smile, believing in it more and more now herself as she went back to her thoughts.

A couple of hours later the Jeep came to a stop. She heard, Stephanie say, "Honey wake up, we're here," shaking Susan's shoulder.

"Oh no, I'm so sorry to have fallen asleep on you," Susan said, wiping the sleep from her eyes. "I cannot believe I did that; I have not fallen asleep in a vehicle since before the accident years ago."

"That's quite all right, I kind of liked it. I now know you trust me, well at least when I drive anyway," she added with a wink. You know that is a very good feeling," Stephanie said kissing the tip of Susan's nose. "Lets get in before you catch a cold," she could feel Susan shivering under her arms.

"It sure is cold out tonight isn't it?" she said shivering again, "you need to take me in and warm me up quickly," Susan added with a smile.

......................................................................................

Tiffany tossed and turned all night, remembering all of Larry's words. Knowing she could never love him the way he should be loved, but knowing she loves him more now for his honesty than ever before. He cared enough about me to be honest with me when I couldn't even be honest with myself Tiffany kept thinking. She also knew even though it hurt she needed to let Susan go, let her be happy even if it was with someone else, she really deserved to be happy at last.

"Easy words to say, now I just need to find the strength in me to live them," Tiffany thought. "Maybe I should get away for a few days." As she drifted off to sleep she knew going away was the best thing she could do for a little while.

"Good morning sunshine," Tiff's mother called out as she came into the house. "Hey now what is all this?" her mother asked as she saw the suitcases sitting by the door.

"Mom, I really need to get away for a few days. I lay wide-awake most of the night thinking about it as well as everything else, and I know it is the best thing to do. I know it will help me clear my head. I called Larry first thing this morning to ask if he would mind if I used one of the tickets we have."

"But those were for the honeymoon," her mother interrupted, "do you think that is appropriate? Using the ticket like that for this reason."

"Mother, at this point I do not know what is or isn't appropriate about anything anymore. He said he didn't mind at all, and that he thinks it is a good idea. I need to go, I've got to Mom."

Mable took Tiffany into her arms as she began to cry, "Honey what is it, why are you so upset?"

"I lost her mom," Tiffany cried, "I really lost her. The bad part is all the years I had her I didn't want her, now I want her and she is gone. What I did was so horrible, I got to make it right and let her go so she can be happy."

"Oh, I am so sorry honey," was all the comfort words Tiffany needed to hear to cause her to break completely down in tears.

At the airport Tiffany promised to call when she got there and got settled in, she wasn't sure how long she would be staying on holiday. She told her mother that she was going to play it by ear and just see. She waved, as her mother pulled away from the curb honking the horn.

"Here you go, you have forty-five minutes until you board," the lady behind the counter said as she handed Tiffany her boarding pass and passport back.

"I sure envy you, I am so tired of this snow, and some sun and sand would be great not to mention another country."

"Not me, I love the snow I just need to get away," Tiffany said as she walked away.

-------------------------------------------------------------------------
-----

"I cannot believe you let me sleep in this late," Susan said after a huge stretch. "Thank you for the snuggling last night not once did I get chilly." I would almost kill for a cup of coffee though, if I didn't need to go out in this nasty white stuff to do it, she added with a giggle.

"I'll go you one better," Steph said laughing also. "For just one little kiss, no chopping or manual labor included, I will pour you a nice big steaming cup."

"Wow, you drive an easy bargain," Susan laughed. "And since you twisted my arm, come here woman, but you know you could have had the kiss without the bribe," Susan teased. "I like it this way too, I get my coffee and your lips," she whispered as she leaned in for a nice long kiss. "I feel at peace here, I hope you know that. I am not big on the cold, wet, white stuff outside, but it too has its fringe benefits. I especially like the cuddling by the fire that I know is to come."

"Oh you think you know this, do you?" Stephanie said. "Just when is this supposed cuddling going to happen, do you figure?"

"Well, if I calculate correct, in about eight hours. It will be dark and even colder out, and I will need to be warmed up," she added with a wink, "or do you think it is just my wishful thinking?"

"Hum, I guess it could be your wishful thinking, but somehow I don't buy it. I do think if I had half the mind to do it I could help you be correct," Stephanie said with a wink.

"Well do you have half the mind?" Susan said when Stephanie didn't finish her statement.

"No baby, I have my whole mind and body wanting to," she added, "now come on, grab your coat and hat, I put some in the bathroom for you to wear."

"Why do I need them, where are we going this early?" Susan asked almost in a playful whine.

"No questions honey just come on, it's a surprise."

"You're a total nut, woman," Susan said as she came into the kitchen bundled up with Steph's things on. "What are you doing? It is the middle of the winter outside, and you're packing a picnic lunch. You have flipped, but I still love ya." Realizing what she had just said, she hurriedly said, "Come on before I roast in all this stuff."

"Hey," Stephanie said. As Susan looked from underneath her cap, Stephanie walked up to her and kissed her right on the eye.

"I love you too Susan, no sorrys, remember? Now lets get out of here girlfriend."

Well into the walk, Susan knew she could go no further.

"I am sorry to say this Steph, but I think I am about to start whining if you don't tell me how much further, I am all tuckered out, when do you think we will be there?"

"Now come on," Steph said. "We don't have that much further to go and no questions remember, you can make it?"

"Well, I do have to admit it is one of the most beautiful places I think I have ever been to."

"Well, my dear Susan, if you think this is pretty just wait until we get there, and then I promise you a sight you will not soon forget. The very best part of it is I get to share it with you."

# CHAPTER 27

After a few more minutes Susan heard Stephanie say, "Hey baby, guess what? We're here."

As they rounded a bend Susan could see why Steph would love this place, it was magical to say the least. There was a huge clearing on the top of the mountain the 360-degree view was spectacular. She felt as if she was on top of the world.

"This is awesome, I am so glad you shared this with me. I am sorry I whined, it was well worth the long hike," she was walking around in circles trying to take in the whole view.

"I know you're cold, but let's have our lunch and talk, ok Susan?"

"That's the funny part, I am not cold at all," she said.

After they had eaten Stephanie began, "when I was a little girl I use to come up here and just sit and dream about everything. To me, there was no better place in the world. After my parent's died, I didn't want anything to do with it any more, none of it at all, not the mountains, not the people, not even the view. It was all reminders; I blamed the mountains. For a long time I would not even come back to this state, and if it wasn't for Miss Rose I would not have ever came back I don't think. The last few days have been one of the hardest times in my life outside of my parent's death, for me to deal with. I believe Susan you were brought to me to be here for me and with me, to help me and to let me help you. I cannot explain how or why this has all happened. I know enough though to know not to question and just to love. I know this may seem rushed and in most cases it would be. I do believe we have both waited our whole life for this, and now that it is here I know I do not want to lose you as I almost did the other day and I know I do not want to wait. It has only been a very short time since we met, but it is a very life long love I feel for you. I will understand if it is too sudden, Susan I am asking you if you will please be with me for life. Be my lover, my life, and my wife."

Stephanie didn't know what hit her as Susan grabbed her, "I love you and all I know thus far about you and I would be honored to spend our lives together. I too believe I was meant to find you, or you find me which ever the case may be. Yes it is fast, but for some reason love doesn't seem to know how to tell time, so to answer your questions. Yes, Yes, Yes," Susan said as she hugged Steph even tighter, crying tears of joy (this time), "Yes I will marry you."

As Steph got down on one knee Susan started giggling.

"Ok," Stephanie said trying to be serious, "I don't have a speech but I want to say this. I don't have a ring to give you right now only my heart. I don't have a song to sing for you only my love. I don't know any of your wishes to grant you, I only have me and all you can see and much, much more."

"You continue to touch my heart with your words even now," Susan began, "I don't need a ring as long as I have you, and I have the song in my heart to sing since I have you and my wish has all ready been granted. You're here, and as for all I can see, well all I can see now is you, my love."

"Susan," Stephanie began, "a few days ago I buried one of the most important people to me, and the same day I found out some news that I need to share with you. You and I need to make some decisions, some very important ones. Robert, the town's one and only lawyer, had handled my parent's will as well as Miss Rose's will now. Susan, Miss Rose was a very wealthy woman more so than even I knew about, and she left it all to me. I brought you up here to show you our mountain, she left this and much more to us."

"Have you given any thought to what you want to do with all this?" Susan asked, looking around, feeling a bit overwhelmed.

"No, I have not thought much about it, I have thought of little else but you darling. I was going to find you if I had to go to Florida and search the Keys alone, now that you're here we will decide together," she added with a smile.

Looking around once more Susan took Steph's hand, "lets go, I'll make some hot cocoa and we can cuddle by the fire and talk. Besides I'm freezing out here now, I think my butt as well as my feet are frozen off."

"You are a big baby," Stephanie said laughing, "I know a way to warm both of them up," she said with a wink. "I love you anyway, big baby or not. Lets go. I'll race you."

"Oh no you don't," Susan said. "I will get lost out here and you will need to come to my rescue yet again, this time I may freeze to death first. I am sticking to you like glue my dear."

"Oh, I must say I do like the sound of that," Steph chipped in.

"It is a much easier walk coming back down the mountain than it is going up," Susan said as they got to the front yard, both out of breath a little.

"You're telling me, I cannot believe I am out of breath."

Stephanie busied herself stoking the fire while Susan made them some hot cocoa; with the fire at a full blaze Steph had an idea.

"I put some extra marshmallows in your cup," Susan was saying as she came into the room, "but I will..." she stopped in mid word as her eyes adjusted to the semi-dark room, she saw Stephanie standing across the room.

"Well don't just stand there with your mouth open woman," Stephanie said with a sly grin. "Do you always let your woman stand alone naked by the fire? Put that chocolate down there and get over here woman, or I might start whining myself."

"Well now, I cannot let you do that, now can I? What kind of woman would I be if I just let you stand there without taking this shirt I have on, off right now? Should I un-button or would you like to?" Susan seductively asked.

"Come here baby," Steph said. "Let me do that for you."

Susan put the cocoa down and slowly walked towards Steph, teasing her a bit as she rubbed her nipples through the fabric of her shirt.

Stephanie slowly started un-buttoning Susan's shirt as she stood in front of her. "I love a woman in flannel, but I sure will like it off you much better."

Hearing Susan moan softly as her fingers brushed the skin under the shirt buttons was more than Stephanie could stand. She ripped the last few buttons off, exposing her right breast a little bit.

"You're beautiful, I never want this moment to end, I will love you forever. Baby with the fire flickering behind you the way it is, I want to make love to you, I need you."

"It seems like it has been forever since we met, and I have wanted you to touch me," Susan groaned as Stephanie's mouth found its way to her neck.

# CHAPTER 28

"Shhh," Stephanie said.

Susan's moans grew louder as Stephanie started sucking on her lips making Susan want even more. She moved on down her neck, lightly kissing and tasting every inch she came to, as Stephanie neared her breast Susan could stay standing no more.

As Susan sat down, she pulled Stephanie down with her, kissing her with a hunger that had been building inside for days. Taking control she heard Steph say, "Oh my God baby this is wonderful, you're wonderful, and it's been so long."

Susan stopped for a minute and pulled back, "No baby," she whispered, "It has been never. This is our time now."

"Yes, yes," Steph responded pulling Susan's head back to her breast. Susan was lightly sucking on each nipple at first, when she could stand it no more Stephanie urged her to suck harder.

"More baby," she pleaded, "harder, oh yes, mmm like that."

As Susan sucked harder on Steph's nipples, she let her hand run over Steph's body, feeling her rock back and forth with desire beneath her. She made sure to save certain spots for later.

Every time Stephanie went to touch Susan or pull her into her even more Susan pulled back as she grabbed her hands and jerked them over her head. This time she used one of her hands to hold Steph's hands in place over her head as her licking and sucking grew more demanding.

"Damn, my skin is on fire," Stephanie whispered. "Please touch me, oh God, please touch me baby. I want to feel you in me, I can't wait baby, please!" she cried out, "fuck me now!"

Susan looked up at Stephanie as the need and hunger grew in her as well. The look of wanting and needing in Steph's eyes driving Susan on.

"I don't want to miss an inch, I will make every inch of you mine before the night is over," Susan emphasized by moving down Steph's body, trailing her lips lightly down her body coming to rest on her stomach and hips. Susan placed her hands on Steph legs to push them open.

She teased the skin on the inside of each leg with her tongue, Steph was shaved all the way and this drove Susan on fast. As her tongue moved closer she felt shivers run through Steph's body and then she cried out, "Please baby, now!" Steph pleaded.

Hearing her pleas Susan took Steph into her mouth.

"Don't stop baby, don't stop!" Stephanie pleaded, afraid Susan was just teasing her again. "Oh God, that feels so great don't ever stop." Hearing Steph's cries only drove

Susan further and faster, she was beginning to feel a quiver grow inside herself.

After the jerks coming from deep within her body had subsided Stephanie pushed Susan off her and onto her back, "I can't wait," Steph groaned, "I've got to have you now," she demanded. As her mouth got to each nipple, she stopped only long enough to kiss one then the other breast, before making her way down Susan's body.

"I feel more alive right now than I ever have," Susan whispered.

As her mouth got to Susan's hot, wet pussy she could wait no more. She pulled open Susan's lips and began sucking and running her teeth and tongue over her, tasting her for the first time, knowing it would not be the last.

"Oh baby, hearing your moans and feeling your soft skin and tasting you has driven me to the brink!" Steph groaned out, "I can't stop," she said. As she rocked her body at the same pace, her fingers moved from Susan's breast to her own pussy. She touched herself as she knew she would explode soon, she knew she was right there. As the movement intensified she took her fingers out of herself and ran them up Susan's leg and deep into her. Susan cried out just as she slammed her fingers back and forth inside her, never stopping the sucking she was doing.

"Oh God baby, I'm going to cummm!!!" Susan said gasping the words out now, "faster oh God baby, faster, oh yes; that's it, that's fucking it. Don't stop! Don't stop!" She grabbed onto Steph's hand pushing her even further into her, needing her as deep as she could go.

Stephanie fucked her faster with her fingers and mouth, holding onto her as tight as she could. She felt her own body explode along with Susan's before collapsing on top of her.

As the fire inside them died down, they just lay by the fire, neither saying a word; there were no words that needed to be said, they both felt a contentment they had not felt before, they didn't need to talk tonight they would talk tomorrow.

Susan had not been this relaxed in a long time. She had forgotten how good sex was, in so many different ways. This time was different though. Sex with other people now seemed so different, even surreal. Stephanie made Susan feel as if she was the only person in the world, or at least the only person that mattered.

They drifted off to sleep as they both watched the fire burn itself low. Susan woke up early, stiff and cold. The fire had died and even the embers were no longer red, they were no more than ash now.

"I am pretty lucky," Susan thought as she watched Steph sleep and seeing her jerk, possibly from a dream she was having. She sat there for a minute more staring at the wisps of hair around Stephanie's delicate forehead. Being careful not to wake her, she got up to grab a blanket off the rocker, as she laid it across Steph she stirred a bit before rolling over, still sound asleep.

As Susan walked over to the window seat in the little alcove off the living room, thoughts of long ago came flooding back. As she was looking out the window at the snow it just brought all the horrible memories of that long ago snowy night back when she was barely seventeen.

"You're evil and disgusting, get out of my house. You have demons in you!" she could remember her Dad screaming that at the top of his voice at her. Her Mother had told her this would happen, but Susan some how didn't believe her. He was strict and mean but never would he do this to his only daughter. Her mother had warned her that as soon as she told her father she was a lesbian he would go nuts.

Now all she could do was just sit on the couch while he screamed at her. He would not even give her time to grab her coat as he threw her out of the house for good. He didn't even care that it was snowing and freezing cold out. As she went out the door, the last words she ever heard him say was that she was vile and sick and a disgrace to him and that he wanted her to burn in hell.

She had grown up in pretty much a poor and rough house. She had three older brothers that did nothing but pick on her, she being the baby and only girl offered her nothing. Her father was a very strict man, not only because he was a preacher but also because his father had raised

177

him that way, the same as his father before him. She never knew the story as to why her oldest brother killed himself when she was just eleven, they told her she was too young to know and from then on her Mother did little else but cry all the time.

It was not until the night she told her Mother that she was in love with Ashley, a girl from school and that they planned on going to college together that she found out the reason her brother committed suicide. She was only seventeen at the time but she felt bold now that she was in love. Her mother felt it was time to tell her all about what had happened with David.

"About a week before he died," her mother began, "your father walked into David's room when David thought he was the only one home. Your father had come home early and caught him...he caught him in bed with a boy," her mother whispered.

"Your father was enraged and he beat them both up badly. He told David that he was sick and awful and that he wished he were dead. You know David was always your father's favorite, he was his first born after all, and he even had hoped that he would follow in his steps and go into the church and take it over one day. Him being gay was just something your father could not accept. It was a week later when I came home from work and found your father sitting in the living room. You were as white as a ghost, sitting there, holding a gun, and crying. Your father said you came home from school right about the time he heard the shot go off in David's room. By the time he got to his room you were already in there screaming. Then you tried to make him wake up, before picking the gun up and going to sit in the living room to watch your father pray."

"I don't remember any of that. All I remember is I came home from school and heard a loud bang. I saw dad come out of David's room, he went right to the living room and got on his knees and started praying. Then, I remember you crying when you got home and at the funeral daddy saying David was in hell because he was evil and that he was a sick person."

"He tells it different, but it is best that you don't remember I'm sure. I think your father blamed himself for your brother some how. He thought the devil was trying to get to him through his kids. And Susan, he will not like what you are going to tell him. Maybe you should just not tell him at all."

"No!" Susan snapped, "I will not lie or hide anymore, we have lived a lie for way too many years here, all of us pretending everything is all right at home and it isn't. I will not live a lie now; I will not spend the rest of my life pretending to be someone I am not just to make him happy. He doesn't care if we are happy so why should we care if he is? I am done being scared of him, I leave in a few months for college, and I will not let him control me any longer as he has all these years. I hate him and I hate this place. When I leave I will never come back here. I don't know why you stay mother, why you let him hit you and hurt us kids in all the ways he does. I hate you too for letting him." That was the last thing her mother ever heard her say to her.

It had gotten really bad that night when she told him about Ashley, he was screaming and she was screaming back. But it was when she told him that she knew what really happened that day with David and that was the reason he hated her so much and that if she had to she would tell, that he screamed.

"Get out and don't you ever come back!" her father spat at her as he grabbed hold of her and threw her out in the snow.

"You're a fag and a queer!" her other brother added.

What hurt Susan the most was that her mother had not even taken up for her; she just sat there on the couch crying and blowing her nose and didn't say a word.

Having no place to go and no way to go anywhere, Susan went to her girlfriend's house. As the door opened and Ashley's dad came to the door she knew something was wrong by the expression on his face.

"Hello Mr. Botts, may I please talk to Ashley?"

"No, she cannot come to the door. She told me about you, and you are no longer welcome here. She cannot talk to you ever again! I will not let a fagot like you ruin my daughter 's life. Now go away and don't you ever dare come back again."

Crying, cold and scared Susan walked back down the drive. She saw Ashley standing at her window, watching her leave. Susan could not tell if she was crying also but when she saw Susan looking at her she shut the curtains and turned out the light. Susan knew that was the end of that. In one hour her whole life had changed forever.

# CHAPTER 29

Susan shivered from her memories as much as from the cold. She hated it when she had the flashbacks like that. They seemed to hit her out of the blue, and it hurt her at times to not know whatever happened to her family. She had grown used to it over the years. She had never told anyone at all, and she didn't think she would ever be able to even tell Stephanie.

"A penny for your thoughts," Stephanie said.

Susan jumped; not knowing Stephanie had woke up. "How long have you been awake?" she asked.

"Actually for a few minutes, I've been lying over here watching you sitting over there. You were deep in thought, which is why I asked what you were thinking about. Nothing bad I hope," Stephanie said.

"No, of course not," Susan fibbed as she gave her a fake smile. "I just woke up early and didn't want to bother you, you were looking so sweet sleeping there and I sometimes wake early. I must say the snow is beautiful this time of the morning; it doesn't even look cold and dirty from in here. It is good thinking and day dreaming time," she added. "Would you like for me to make us some coffee?" Susan said as she unwrapped her legs from under herself to get up.

"Sounds great, I think I will go have a nice long shower, I feel sticky this morning," Stephanie said embarrassed with her own comment. "Hey, next time you better wake me," she added as she headed to the bathroom.

"Yes, next time," Susan thought, knowing there would be many next times. The dreams and memories were coming now more frequently than ever before.

As Susan made the coffee a smile crossed her lips as her mind once again filled with memories. This time they were not of so long ago, Susan had never had this feeling of togetherness before, not even with Tiffany.

Stephanie was so easy to talk to she thought about telling her all about her past. She wanted to share it with her, but was afraid in doing so that she may just bore her to death or make her want to run for the hills.

All Susan had from her life before was her memories and stories. Though mostly bad ones, they still help make up who she was now, so she wondered if she should tell her. Before now she had not had anyone to share them with. The best thing now was that she was going to have new stories to tell, so why keep the old ones locked away anymore. She decided when the time was right, she would tell her everything.

"Even though she had only known Stephanie for a little while there were several new tales to tell already, well to at least replace the old bad ones," she thought with a smile.

In a way everything seemed like a dream. After all, it is not everyday that you fall in love with a wonderful woman in such a short amount of time and become the owner of a mountain!

Susan had some apprehension about that one; not that owning a mountain was bad, but because of the location of the mountain. Susan had gotten away from this part of the country for a reason a long time ago, now she was being pulled back to it and she wondered why.

She was not sure at all how she was going to handle it, Stephanie was so excited about it and she loved Colorado. Susan knew that she had to be strong during this time; she certainly did not want to do anything to jeopardize her and Steph's relationship. What did it really matter where they lived?

Susan also knew that she had to be true to herself, could she deal with the stress of moving back to Colorado after all she had gone through before? Of course, it was not the mountains fault but all the memories of the past were at times still very vivid in her mind. Especially since she had been back in this state, as if it was only yesterday that the awful occurrences of her childhood had taken place.

Certain places trigger memories, even certain smells she knew. That was one thing about Key West that she loved, the scent of wood burning in fireplaces is very rare there. The feel of salt-water condensation on ones skin is what Susan loves the most about Key West, it was the farthest feeling from cold snow and mean people she could get. She didn't get the same bad dreams and flashbacks in Florida as she found she was getting here in the Rockies.

Things had been moving so fast, Susan wondered how it was that people's feelings about others could change so much in such a short period of time. One week you dislike a person and then the next you like them and dislike someone you have liked before.

It was not that Susan and Tiffany had developed a dislike for one another; they just had differing feelings about what it meant to be in love and need someone and also what the lesbian lifestyle was all about and all that it meant to be gay.

Susan knew that deep in her heart, she would always love Tiffany, and part of her would anyway. She wasn't sure why she had held on to the hope of them getting back together for so long, when she knew there was no hope left. She knew that moving on now was the right thing to do. She just could not live her life in a vacuum, trying to avoid all the negative ramifications of the homosexual lifestyle that some tried to make you believe was there. She never believed it at all, to her there was nothing wrong with her or how she lived and loved. She didn't know why she was thinking of Tiffany at all right now, but hearing the coffee pot percolate jarred Susan back to the sounds of Stephanie in the shower singing away.

"Coffee's ready, get your fine ass out of the shower my lady," she yelled out to Stephanie.

"I feel much better now," Steph said as she came out of the shower in nothing but a towel, "I am thinking of not putting any clothing on today at all," she whispered into Susan's ear. Coming up behind her she kissed the back of Susan's neck as she ran her hands under Susan's shirt that she had on to rub her nipples. The shirt was the only thing she had bothered to put back on, and Stephanie wished she had not bothered with any clothing at all.

Susan closed her eyes and leaned back against Stephanie as she continued to rub and squeeze her nipples. As Susan purred into Steph's ear, she decided to explore further she ran her other hand down her stomach and between her legs, she didn't have her panties on so Stephanie cupped her hand over Susan; letting her fingers push into her, massaging as she went. She could feel Susan's wetness already, hot and sticky, as she let her fingers slip in through her slit, it only took a few strokes of her fingers until Susan started bucking against her as she started moaning and jerking wildly.

"Damn baby, I like the sound of that," Stephanie said as she pumped harder, "cummm for me baby," she demanded. As she gave her nipple another hard squeeze, Susan cried out with pleasure calling Stephanie's name. Then Steph ran that hand down her back to cup her ass in her hand, she slowly teased her ass before letting one of her fingers slip into Susan's asshole, very slowly and gently she started pumping with both her hands now filling Susan up. After a few minutes more Susan started bucking wildly into Stephanie's fingers.

"Fuck me!!" she was screaming, "fuck me!!" As Susan let her body convulse then stop she exhaled loudly as she turned around to kiss Steph. With tears of passion and satisfaction in her eyes, she whispered, "I love you baby," into Steph's mouth along with the kisses.

Susan could smell the aroma of their lovemaking and she wanted Stephanie badly, as she reached out for her Steph stopped her. "Go shower, I am not through with you just yet, I'll reheat the coffee."

"I think I may run around like this also today," Susan said after her shower coming into the kitchen naked except for the towel wrapped around her hair, "but my butt might get too cold," she added.

"Not if I keep it warm for you, did I tell you I was an ass woman?" she added a bit embarrassed.

Stephanie giggled when Susan said, "good because that's one thing I just found out I liked," she said with a huge smile.

As Stephanie finished re-heating the coffee, she poured two cups full for them both. Susan decided to try and get the fire going. Coming back into the kitchen she said, "hey, where is all the wood? How am I going to make a fire with wet wood?"

"Honey, there is plenty of wood in the wood box, did you check in there? Come on, I will show you," she offered as she saw the confused look on her face.

Feeling like a real heal, Susan let Stephanie lead her into the living room to show her where the wood is kept.

She tried to play it off with, "I knew that all along," Susan attempted to make Stephanie believe, "but I don't want to hurt your pride so I'll let you make the fire."

Stephanie had to laugh out loud with that one.

"What?" Susan pouted. "Why are you making fun of me?"

"Come here honey," Steph said as she hugged Susan, "I would never make fun of you much, anyway," she added, "and I am no God or a match stick by any means. I don't make fire but I will start a fire for you baby girl," she added with a smile and a wink. "You know I love picking at you?"

"Well I never…" Susan began.

"I can see that! Just by the way you tried to start this fire," Stephanie cut in with a laugh.

"Stop it, see your doing it again, be good," Susan said with a love tap to Steph's arm.

"Oh, I am going to get you for that one," Stephanie snickered, as she ran after Susan who took off dropping the towel as she went.

"I sure hope so," Susan said as she ran from Stephanie.

# CHAPTER 30

Stephanie caught up with her at the stairway, "I got you," she yelled with a giggle, "and whatever I got is very soft and squishy," she squealed.

"Oh you sure did, or did I let you get me?" Susan said as she sat down on the bottom step.

"Oh no you don't, I caught you fair and square," she said as she leaned down for a long wet kiss.

"Well, for a kiss like that you can catch me any time," pulling Stephanie down with her she nuzzled her ear.

Then Stephanie started trailing little kisses down Susan's shoulder causing her to shiver. Pulling back she looked deep into Steph's eyes. Before she had a chance to say anything Susan took her mouth forcefully, all during her shower she could still feel Steph's hands on her and in her.

"I have got to have you right now," she whispered into Steph's breasts, sucking on each.

"Don't you want to go up to the bed?" Stephanie purred.

For the answer Susan's mouth and tongue found the wet spot between her legs. Refusing to move, she would not lick her clit yet, all she would do was blow on it, making Stephanie shiver with lust.

Stephanie tried to push her head down; she had to feel her mouth on her. When that didn't work she tried to arch her ass upwards, bucking into Susan's mouth.

Susan grabbed on to Steph's hips and pinned her down. "I will fuck you when I am ready, right now be still," she demanded with a smile on her lips, Stephanie dropped her ass and obeyed Susan.

"I am in charge right now and you will do as I say," she said with so much lust in her voice that her words came out raspy. She could see what and how she was saying things was turning Stephanie on even more.

As she stood up and moved back from Stephanie she pulled her up with her. As Stephanie was about to speak Susan told her to shut up. She led her to the living room and sat her down on the floor. As she sat down across from her, she spread her legs.

"Now do not move," she commanded, "do not even take your eyes off me. "Susan reached down and took one of her own nipples between her fingers and started squeezing it, she arched her hips a bit to make sure Stephanie could get a good look at her pussy, she then slowly ran her other hand down her stomach. She let her hand linger over her belly before traveling on down, she could see Stephanie watching her every move. She slowly let one finger slip into her wetness, then another and another, as she started moving her hips and fingers faster it was all Stephanie could do to not move as she started shifting her weight. Once

190

Susan began moaning, Stephanie started licking her lips and pleading with her eyes.

"Not yet," Susan whispered between gasps of breath.

As she grew very close to the edge, she looked over to Stephanie saying, "Now baby, now, fuck yourself for me. I want to see your fingers touching yourself. Don't say anything, just do it. Oh yes baby, that's it, faster," she demanded, "faster, oh yes, yes, that's it." She could see that Stephanie was close now and as she reached down and began fucking herself again they both screamed out at the same time, watching one another was all it took to put them both over the edge.

They spent most of the morning making love and fucking. In the tub Stephanie took control and fucked Susan that time and then on the floor and in the bed they made love.

As the sun was setting, Stephanie sat up in bed, "So do you want to go into town and get some dinner? For some reason I am hungry, we can sit and have a drink with dinner and talk. I know we only have a couple more days before you need to head back, and I would like to talk things over first, maybe make some lasting plans."

"Sounds great," Susan agreed. "I am ravenous I have sure worked up an appetite today," she added with a wink.

It had taken them quite a while to get ready, after they showered together and was about to head out the door Susan stopped in the hall and turned to Stephanie.

"You know dear, it would not have taken us as long to get going," Susan said as they were about ready to leave, "if you had been able to keep your hands off me in the shower."

"Well now that is just too bad isn't it? I like my hands on you," Stephanie said as she slowly ran her hands over Susan to show her she meant business. "If we didn't need to go eat to stay alive I would not let you out of this house for as long as I could keep you here."

As they were going out the door Susan stopped dead in her tracks, remembering that she had made a deal with herself to tell Stephanie a little bit at least before they left. "Stephanie, before we go I need to tell you something."

"You're not going to quarrel at me again for wanting to touch you are you?" Then seeing the look on Susan face she became worried. "What is it honey, is something wrong?"

"I have not told you very much about my past and I am sorry. I just feel like I need to tell you this before we go. When I was small we lived here in Colorado, but it was a really bad life and it was one I never wanted to remember so I put it out of my mind and didn't ever want to remember it. No one knows, not even Tiffany. It's just something I never thought or talked about but I felt you needed to know at least a little of why I am not big on being in this state, I don't want to bore you to death," she added, "but if you want to know anything just ask ok and with time I am sure I will be telling you more."

"Thank you for sharing with me what you feel you can honey, you have your reasons and I understand. I want you to know baby that you can tell me anything. I will never judge you and I will always be here for you, but I don't want you to tell me before you are ready to, I can and will wait."

"I know," Susan said. "That is just a part of me I don't want to remember, but for some reason since I have been here it keeps coming back to me. The first night I was here when you woke to find me asleep on the couch it was because of a dream I had. I saw in your eyes the next morning that you thought it was because of Tiffany but it wasn't."

"That's where your mind was and what you were thinking about when I woke up this morning wasn't it? I saw you sitting over at the window lost in your own world."

"Yes that was where my mind was," Susan answered. "I don't mean to exclude you and I will get better I promise. I have not had anyone to share things with like that before. I even wondered if I would tell you at all but I knew I had to. Thank you for understanding and for just being there," Susan added. "Now let's go eat, before I starve to death."

"The sun must have shined quite a bit today," Stephanie remarked, "there are clear patches on the road. I know it didn't snow at all today, not that I got much of a chance to see outside," she added with a sly smile, "oh and did I say thank you for today?"

"No thanks needed," Susan whispered.

"Is that a blush I see?"

"No," Susan said laughing, "well not much of one anyway. I just hate when I blush, it is so a teen thing to do. I always thought I would grow out of it."

"I like it," Stephanie said with a smile. "I hope you never grow out of it."

As they pulled the Jeep into the parking lot Susan noticed how busy it was.

"I didn't think it would be so busy on a cold night like this. Who in their right minds would go out on an evening like this unless they just didn't have food in the house and had to go out to eat to live," she said with a smile as a jab to Stephanie.

"Heck, this is great weather for this time of year; I am surprised we can find a place to park at all, oh and I forgot to tell you," Stephanie added, "tonight is karaoke night."

"Oh no. Don't you even think you are going to get me to sing a song. Nope, nope, nope never ever! I would pass right out, so no way," Susan added to make sure Stephanie got the point.

They only had to wait about ten minutes to get a table, and after they were seated Susan remarked, "This sure is a busy little place isn't it? It is really nice," Stephanie, "thank you for bringing me here."

"This is one of my most favorite places when I am in town, they have great food and drinks and I think the thing I like the most is the people. You'll see what I mean before the night is over."

They had been at their table no more than a few minutes when a gentleman walked over.

"Evening Sheriff," Stephanie said, "I would like you to meet my girlfriend, Susan. Susan, this is Sheriff Knox."

"Nice to meet you Mr. Knox," she said as she stuck out her hand to shake his.

He just laughed and grabbed her for a big ole bear hug. "Hey now I'll have none of that Mr. stuff, just call me Sheriff, everyone else does. Have fun tonight ladies and I better get a treat and hear you sing tonight my dear."

"Oh now," Susan cut in, "I don't sing, that is not my cup of tea but thank you anyway."

He just smiled as he turned to Stephanie and said after he kissed her on the cheek, "I'm here for you if you need me. It's good to see you out and about, Miss Rose would have wanted that." Then he leaned over and whispered something in Stephanie's ear that Susan could not make out. Stephanie just laughed and shook her head as if to say yes and then she winked at him.

After he left the table Susan turned to Stephanie saying, "Boy he sure is friendly, he caught me off guard. So are you going to tell me what he whispered? You know that's rude," she said with a smile she was trying to guilt Stephanie into telling her.

"I will not tell you," she said with a smile, "anyway you will see. As for the people, you will get use to it in no time," Stephanie said, "Everyone is just like that in this town, it really is like one big family."

After they gave their dinner orders to the waitress Stephanie excused herself to go to the bathroom. Susan felt relaxed sitting and listening to the little old bald guy belting out "Ain't Nothin' But A Hound Dog" by Elvis Presley. She could have sworn that he didn't have a tooth in his head.

"It is nice to see you smiling like that darling," Stephanie remarked as she got back to the table.

"Well I am happy but I must confess that I find that most humorous," she said, as she looked towards the stage as the little old guy finished his song. "I don't know why in the world anyone would ever want to get up in front of a room full of people and bark out songs. I like to listen and watch other people but I would just die if I ever had to, I have stage fright so bad, and I don't think anyone sounds good doing karaoke anyway."

"We'll see," Stephanie said with a sneaking grin.

Just as Susan was about to ask Stephanie what she meant she was stopped dead in mid-sentence as the waitress brought their drinks out, and two more people carrying their food out followed her.

Susan had forgotten all about Stephanie's remark, as she tasted her food." Wow this is wonderful," Susan said taking a big bite.

# CHAPTER 31

"Next up," the announcer said interrupting the rest of Susan's enjoyment of her food when she heard. "We have Susan joining Stephanie this time tonight; they're going to sing "I Honestly Love You" By Olivia Newton- John. Lets all give them a big round of applause."

Susan had just put what felt like was a huge bite into her mouth when the spotlights hit them. She knew her cheeks were bulging out.

Half choking out, more with pleading eyes than words, "NO, NO, NO," but Stephanie was having none of it as she grabbed Susan's arm and drug her up to the stage.

"Come on and live a little," Stephanie was saying, "I do this all the time, you will love it. No one will care how good or bad you are," she added. "And you might want to swallow that food or you might spit it out onto the people in the front row while you're singing," she said laughing.

"But, but, but... Susan felt like a deer caught in the headlights. With nowhere to go except stand there and get hit or give in as the case may be.

Stephanie said, "Just have fun. We all get up here sooner or later."

"Pleeease let mine be later," Susan begged.

"No way, it's our turn."

"I cannot carry a tune," Susan pleaded, "not even if I had a huge bucket to carry it in."

As the music started Stephanie grabbed the microphone and started singing, "I love you...I honestly love you..."

Stephanie handed Susan the microphone right at the same time as she groaned out loud, "Oh God."

"Oh, I'll get you for this," she whispered to Stephanie as all the people clapped and laughed having heard what she said yet again.

"You can do it!" she heard someone shout out in the audience.

"I mean I'll get you big time," she said as her part to sing came up.

"Come on and join us," she heard Stephanie say as the music was playing, a huge sigh of relief came over Susan knowing no one would be able to hear her while she sounded as if someone was killing the cat.

"You're not singing, you're lip-syncing," Stephanie said to the back of her head as the crowd sang at the top of their lungs.

"They will never know the difference!" Susan yelled back at Stephanie.

After the song was over, they made their way back to the table. Susan was relieved it was over and that she didn't pass out. Stephanie was just happy that she had gotten her up on stage at all.

"That was great babe, thank you for doing it for me. Your not to mad at me are you? Lets finish dinner then we can talk, ok Susan?"

"Hell yes I am mad at you," she said, "and I didn't do it for you, I had no choice in it," she added the giggle so Stephanie would know she was just joking.

Dinner had been good and so much fun. Susan had not had this much fun in a long time, she could not believe she actually got up and did karaoke in front of everyone. Now it was time for them to sit down and decide what they were going to do with the rest of their lives together, or at least for now Susan thought.

There was an uneasy feeling in Susan's stomach. She was not looking forward to this discussion. She had not talked with Stephanie much about her past and she was not sure that Steph would understand or even still want her if she knew how bad it had been. She said she understood but would she still if she knew it all?

"So where do we begin?" Stephanie asked Susan. "There are so many decisions to be made and so much to talk about, I have no idea where to even begin."

"Well, we probably need to discuss where we are going to live first off, we both have said we want to be together now we figure out where," Susan said. "I don't mean to be like this, but I really do love Florida, the sand and the ocean air and the heat. It is so far away from all the bad and it is just home to me, and I know you love the mountains; I think we may have a problem on this one. I think first we need to talk about what you want to do with the land and the mountain and stuff. Then we can talk about the hard one of where to live, what do you think Steph?"

"Well, I agree with you that it will be a decision we both need to make, but it is what we want to do," Steph corrected, "Not just what I want to do with it. OK?"

"But Miss Rose left the land to you sweetheart. It is all yours. Have you thought about all the responsibilities there are to owning property? Have you gone to the tax assessor's office to find out how much property tax is yearly? Have you thought of how you will keep the property up as far as mowing and upkeep?"

"Whoa, slow down on the questions," she said with a smile. "First of all, the mountain is not all that Miss Rose left me, errrr…us," she corrected, "She left a sizable monetary amount also. It will be more than enough to maintain the upkeep and then some so no worries there. She knew I would not be able to take care of things on what I make alone."

"One thing you might want to consider is maybe dividing up the land into plots and selling it off in bits," Susan suggested. "This way you could make money off of it and not have to do anything else with it."

"NO!" Stephanie replied quite angrily. "There is no way that I am selling off the land that way, and we don't need money off it anyway. That is not how Miss Rose would have wanted it. She hated it when developers would come in and destroy wonderful land and forest like that with no consideration for the wild life and plants that live on it. That, my dear, is not a choice."

"I am sorry, I didn't mean to upset you. It's just that you are the one that said it was ours and we were going to talk about it." Susan answered. "I am just trying to come up with ideas of things to do with it, I wasn't aware that you was planning to keep it yourself. Do you have anything in mind yourself?"

"Well, to tell you the truth I do have something in mind. I am sorry I snapped at you, I didn't mean it; I guess it is all still fresh with her dying and all. What she left me is all I have left of her. What would you think about maybe turning part of the land into a commune?"

Seeing the look on Susan's face Steph quickly went on, "I do not mean a man hating woman's group that sits around man bashing and smoking dope all day. I mean a nice place, maybe with some campgrounds so that young men and women, teens even, can come to find answers about themselves. It will be for lesbian and gay people. I feel so lucky to have had Miss Rose as my support system, but if I had not had her I do not know where I would have turned. I know there are a lot of kids out there that have nowhere to turn or no one to turn to at all, and well I have always wanted to mentor to young adults. I know I am not making any sense, please let me know what you are thinking. I know there would be a lot of work getting something like that going but I think you and I could do it, and I think it would be great for this area also. Anything new would bring a lot of needed work and people to this town."

"I agree that it would be a lot of hard work," Susan said. "I like the idea per say but what about more along the lines of a Bed and Breakfast hotel slash campgrounds. We could have a stable also; I believe many people would love to be able to go for a ride before breakfast or at sunset. We could have a little camping area for tents and RVs so if they prefer that over staying in the main house we would have that as a choice. We would need to get some help to run it when we're not here and what all would you want it to offer? The list of questions goes on."

"I think I really do like that idea, it's along the same lines as I was talking about maybe just softer and your way we would reach a lot more people also, not just the gay community," Steph added.

"I had not thought of that, we need to do some research on what we need to get either a commune or B&B going. If we divide up and each take an area to research we will have answers a lot quicker. I really am looking forward to us doing this together," Susan said taking Steph's hand in hers, "who knows this just may be the therapy I was needing to help stop the dreams."

"You may be right," Stephanie said. "I want to do whatever I can to make you happy. I just want us to make the right decisions at the beginning so that we will have no regrets later on down the road, know what I mean?"

Susan nodded her agreement.

# CHAPTER 32

"Dinner was great Stephanie, thank you for bringing me here. I am still not wild about the singing part of it," Susan added, "but the food was great as well as the atmosphere."

"I'm glad you liked it," Stephanie said. "I knew you would," she added with a smile. "Why don't we get some coffee and go out on the porch. We can talk more about these ideas of ours?"

"Are you crazy? It is cold out there," Susan said with a perplexed look on her face.

Laughing, Stephanie just shook her head, "No silly, it is a closed-in porch, they just don't play the music out there so it is quiet and you can sit and talk. There is even couches so it gives it a homey feel, come on I'll show you."

As they received a number for the coffee they had ordered, they went out to the side porch to wait on the waitress to bring it to them.

"Now why in the world do they call this a porch?" Susan wondered out loud. "I like it but it isn't a porch to me."

Stephanie just smiled at Susan.

They both sat there for a minute. "Stephanie, may I ask you a question? Where do you see us in a couple years? Have you given it any thought yet? I know it is all so fast and new still."

"Well," Stephanie began, "I know that we will be together; I hope it is running our own place here in the mountains. I have not ruled out the possibility that it may be somewhere else. There is also so much to learn about one another, and I would like to take time to get to know you and you get to know me also. We have a lot to learn yet, let's not be in a rush. I have thought about one day way in the future adopting a kid also, at least one little one. Of course that will depend on how you feel about children. I love the mountains and I hope we can stay here as I said, I think you could learn to love it here with me, I hope," she added.

"What if I don't learn to love them? And what if I don't want to have kids? Hell with the way I was brought up I'm not even sure I would make a good mother. Don't get me wrong, I have thought of it, but I just don't know. There are so many things we need to talk about. I think we have really jumped in deep without knowing much about the other, don't you think?"

Steph was a bit taken aback with what Susan was now saying.

"First everyone is scared to be a parent the first time and second we are not talking about having one anytime soon and are you having second thoughts already?" Steph challenged.

"No ma'am, I'm not," Susan offered. "It is just questions we have not had the time to ask or to discuss at all with one another. These are life-changing decisions, you know?

What if the mountains are not where I want to move? What if I can't or won't move here, then what? Do we have a then what?"

Stephanie felt a bit cornered. Susan seemed to be trying to pick a fight, "I don't mean to get on the defensive Susan, but I remember you telling me you bought a snow suit and were all but packed and ready to move to Colorado for Tiffany." Then seeing the look on Susan's face, Stephanie hurried to add, "If this is because I tricked you into getting up there and singing..." Stephanie tried to lighten the mood up, "then I am sorry."

"Come on Steph, we need to talk about this. You know I am not mad about that, I am just worried about tomorrow and the next and the next."

"Well stop worrying so much please, as long as we are together then all of our tomorrow's we can get through together," Stephanie added.

"I'm sorry," Susan, answered in a whisper, "we just need to talk it all out is all."

"Ok, I am sorry also, and I agree we do need to talk about this. Do you have any other ideas? Please just jump in and throw them out there, I told you my idea about the commune and I do want to hear more of yours on the B&B. The more I think about it the more I am really liking the idea. I am sorry if I don't seem receptive to your thoughts."

"Well," Susan began, and then she stopped as the waitress brought their coffees out to them.

"Ok where was I?" Susan went on after she left, "OK, first, thank you for that. And as I said, I have always wanted to open a nice quaint Bed and Breakfast, maybe one mostly catering to the lesbian world even, if that would make you feel better," she added, "I was thinking about it having a little coffee shop and maybe a little store in it. I had thought it would be in Florida around the ocean, but I am trying to be open. As for kids I have not given kids much serious thought. My feelings change on that as the season changes at times it seems; I must admit."

Stephanie thought for a minute and said, "You know, the more I think about it the more your idea is really growing on me. I haven't even thought of a B&B before tonight, and you know I like the idea of a lesbian B&B but we do not only have to cater to them. We can be open and friendly to all. As for kids, that is something we can just think about and talk about in time. Who knows we may be too busy to worry about them even," she added. "But I do think the people around here would like the B&B idea really well. It would do so much for the..."

"Around here?" Susan cut in. "I don't know about around here, I was talking more about in Key West. Honey I don't mean to sound negative, I know you don't want to sell and I do understand that. What if we donated part of the land to some worthy causes, not all of it, we could look at living in Florida. Have you ever thought about living at the ocean? Do you even like the ocean?" she added.

"Honestly no, I have not ever thought about moving, I have never even been to Florida nor have I saw any other oceans. I am not big on salt water I guess," Stephanie thought for a few minutes before continuing, "Tell you what, to be fair we can do the research that we need to do anywhere. So how would you like it if I go with you back to Florida when you go, I can see the area and give it a look see? We would have more time to talk about all things. If we decided to move here I would all ready be there to help you pack your things; if we want to be there, then I am there with you to help find us a place."

"You know," Susan said after thinking about it, "I would like that very much. Thank you for giving it some thought, it means a lot to me that you would make that effort."

"I will go you one better even," Stephanie said. "If you would like to try and get a flight out tomorrow we can go then so we won't chance getting snowed in again, it would only be a few days earlier than when you were going to be leaving anyway."

Susan was excited to be going home. "You know what dear? I am happy to be going back but I think I am even happier knowing you are going to go with me, and I think it is a great idea about tomorrow. As I have found out, this weather is something you do not know about from one day to the other. Thank you for thinking about it for me, and I have every confidence that once you get to Florida you will just love it. Just wait and see," she added with a smile.

"Well, come on woman. What are you waiting for? Drink your coffee so we can go pack," Stephanie said with a laugh.

Seeing Stephanie pack only winter clothing she had to laugh, "Honey remember it is not going to be cold there, don't forget to put some summer clothing in also. I am rooting for you to pack the teeny weenie bikini I saw you stuff way back in the back of that drawer you just had open," Susan added with a wink. "At it's coldest it is only 78 degrees and up."

"Wow," Stephanie remarked a little dryly.

"Hey now, don't be so down. You said you was going to give this a shot, if you are upset and mad it will not be a fair shot."

"I know and I am sorry," Stephanie said. "I will try to be better about all this, it isn't that I don't want to go. I do, it is just something new, and you will find out in time that I am not into new things much, so please bear with me."

# CHAPTER 33

"I cannot believe you do not have two seats together," Stephanie snapped at the guy behind the counter, raising her voice she added, "We got here early and sat for two hours, all we want is two seats together. We are a couple together and want to sit together!"

"I am sorry ma'am. I am also sorry you feel the need to shout at me, but we are all full with passengers that saw fit to book a seat before we were about to take off. As I told you before I have only three seats left on the whole plane and none of them are together. You may have gotten here early and sat for a while, but when you do not bother calling ahead and making reservations you get what is left, and you are lucky there is any left. If you have not noticed as of late it is cold here and most people that can are trying to get out of here and Florida to them sounds like a better choice. Now do you want the seats or not?"

"We will take the seats," Susan said as she stepped in front of Stephanie handing him her credit card, taking hold of Steph's hand she lead her aside, "Are you ok honey? This is not like you at all," she added.

"I am just a little edgy is all, I hate flying. I'll be better once we get there, I promise."

The flight went smooth to Susan's relief. Knowing now that Stephanie didn't care to fly, she had grown worried that it may be bumpy with the weather and all. She was glad they got a direct flight even if they could not sit together. Stephanie was on edge enough over this trip and she didn't want to make it worse on her.

As they stepped off the plane all Susan heard Stephanie say was, "Damn it's hot, it's the middle of wintertime and I feel like I cannot even breathe for all this heat."

Trying to lift her mood Susan said, "Hey now, you said you were going to be open minded, stop being a grumpy butt. Let me call Mr. Edwards and see if he could pick us up, be right back," Susan said as she was heading to the phone. A couple of minutes later she returned saying that Mr. Edwards was out until this evening as he didn't know we were coming in a day early, so she ordered a cab be sent to pick them up.

Susan saw Stephanie roll her eyes at the news; she just pretended she hadn't seen it.

As they waited at the airport for the taxi Stephanie asked, "Is the ride to your house a long one?"

"Well, no," Susan said with a smile. "This island isn't that big, it doesn't take long to get anywhere. That is one of the things I love about it."

"Thank God it is here," Stephanie said seeing the cab pull up, "I thought I was going to sweat to death before it even got here."

212

After Susan gave the address both women were pretty quiet on the drive. Susan was just glad to be back, and Stephanie wondered how anyone could live in this humid climate. To make matters worse, the cab didn't even have air conditioning in it. She had to roll her window down, which she found out didn't help any; it only blew warm salt air around making her feel sticky, and in even more of a bad mood.

As the cab came to a stop Stephanie seeing where they were asked, looking around in shock, "Why are we here Susan? I thought we were going to go to your house."

"This is my house Stephanie. I'm sorry I didn't think to tell you."

"Oh you've got to be kidding, please tell me you are kidding," seeing a hurt and shocked look on Susan face she went on quickly, "you mean to tell me that you live in a boat on the water?" A bit disbelieving at it all, Steph was feeling very overwhelmed and it was all she could do to chuck back tears that were ready to spill out. The flight, then the heat and humidity, and the houseboat were just all too much for her right now.

The cabbie just stared at Stephanie as he got the bag out of the trunk, making her feel even worse if that was even possible she thought.

"Come on," Susan said grabbing the bags, "let me show you around and then we can talk about it. Trust me it isn't as bad as it seems, and it is a lot bigger than it looks also, you will see."

"It isn't the size," Stephanie said. "It's just the fact that it is on the water, and I know I am going to get motion sickness again like on the plane. I am not good in the air or on the water. I do not mean to be this way; I am just a land lover I guess. I never would have ever in my wildest dream thought you lived on a boat or I would have said something. I'm sorry, I think it might just be jet lag or something," she offered. "Let me just lay down a bit please, I am sure that a nap will help."

As they boarded the boat a small wave hit and this only made it worse for Stephanie as the boat rocked a little bit. Susan held her breath as she showed Steph where she could rest, hoping that no more waves would be that strong.

Thanking Susan, Steph lay down, she felt worse than if she was on that old waterbed one of her ex's had. She hated it and she hated this now. She didn't think she would be able to fall asleep before getting sick but a little while later after only a short nap Stephanie opened her eyes and just lay there for a minute not realizing where she was. She then felt the motion of the swaying boat and it all came back to her. She could honestly say she was totally wrong, she didn't feel any better at all.

"Hey you, that was a short nap," Susan said as Stephanie came out of the bedroom, "How are you feeling? Any better?" she said hopefully.

"Well to be honest," Stephanie said, "I don't feel much better at all."

"Well just for you I turned the air on full blast, I thought that might help and you're lucky, not too many people down here even have air conditioners. I had the fortitude to have one added when I gave the specs for the boat I wanted since I like it a little cooler in the summer months than most do around here. I also made us a light lunch of some fruit and cheese and crackers, which always seems to help me settle my stomach after a trip. I promise it will get better if you just try and relax," Susan said and then kissed her on the nose, as a mother would do to reassure a child.

As they were sitting on the deck Stephanie started to turn several shades of green right in front of Susan, it was then she decided she couldn't eat anything. Susan knew it was time to pull the medicine out of the closet. It didn't take long for the Dramamine to take effect, "thank goodness," she thought.

After a bit Stephanie opened her eyes and said, "I feel much better now. Show me to my fruit platter, maybe if I get something on my stomach it will help as the Dramamine has made me jittery with nothing to eat all day. I could not even think about food on the plane," she said, trying to offer a tiny smile. Susan appreciated the effort Stephanie was making to not be too grumpy.

To help keep her stomach settled Susan made Stephanie a cup of green tea. Afterwards as Stephanie was trying to sip the tea she decided it was time to start in on the questions. First one, then another, she started with, "So tell me why in the world you would want to live on a boat? Who in their right mind would want to live on one of these things?" she added, "I mean no offense or anything, it just never crossed my mind that anyone would want to. I mean don't get me wrong I knew they did, but why?"

Smiling, Susan said, "No offense taken, I just love the water and the sun and the salt air. I love the motion of the water at night while I sleep as if it is gently rocking me, and I feel like I have a lot of freedom living this way. I can pull up anchor at any time and go at a moments notice. Hey and no grass to cut at all," Susan added with a giggle. "When I first moved here, I rented a small house just up the road, a cottage really, a friend of mine from school has a houseboat and when I would come over for barbeques and get together I just loved it so when my lease was almost up, I decided to custom order this boat and I have loved it ever since," she added.

"Well if you lived in an apartment like sane people do there would be no grass to cut either, so that isn't much of an argument for living here," Stephanie said under her breath, but loud enough for Susan to hear. "The water is really choppy isn't it, is it like this all the time? And is it this hot in the summer also?"

"Most of the time it doesn't get above eighty-two degrees in the summer and no lower than seventy-two degrees in the winter. You will get use to the humidity, as for why it is so choppy, it is hurricane season, nothing for you to worry about, it just makes the water pretty choppy for a few days."

Seeing the look on Steph's face Susan hurried and went on. "There isn't much change in the temperature from one season to the other, the temperature is pretty much the same all year long. We have our wet days and our dry days, we have our cool days and our hot days," Susan was saying, "but we're on a pretty even keel."

Taking Steph's hand in hers she said, "Please give it a couple of days and see how you feel. So much has happened in such a short time, and I want you to like it here. If you don't after you have given it a fair shake then we will talk more about getting a house or hotel or something, ok?"

Stephanie just nodded her ok.

"And to not sound too nasty," she added with a smile. "I want us to make love on the water."

"Well, I don't know about that," Steph said, "I think the boat moved way too much already for that," she said, trying to smile as she leaned over and kissed Susan. She knew Susan was trying to make her feel better, and she knew she was not helping matters any by acting this way.

Their kisses grew more passionate and Susan felt hope that Stephanie was relaxing a little bit. As Stephanie pulled Susan closer deepening her kiss she let her hand run over

Susan's shoulders and down her arm. As her thumb brushed Susan's breast Stephanie felt a tingle run through her. She started fondling Susan's breast as they kissed and could hear Susan moan. She ran her hands over Stephanie they were sitting out on the deck and neither seemed to mind. Stephanie ran her hand under Susan's top and found she didn't have a bra on, this made Steph want to explore more. Taking Susan's nipples between her fingers she caressed and pulled at them as Susan rolled her head back a bit inviting Stephanie to kiss her neck. She felt no shame with Steph at all. As Stephanie started licking and kissing Susan's neck a wave suddenly hit the boat causing Stephanie to pull back quickly.

"Come here baby," Susan said trying to pull Stephanie back to her.

"No I can't right now, I'm sorry baby," Stephanie said. "But my stomach doesn't feel so well again."

Susan was hurt. She didn't feel Stephanie was trying very hard. The wave had not even been a strong one but she decided to drop it, saying, "Well dear, I need to run down the pier for a few minutes to let Mr. Edwards know I am back. I told his partner Ben when I called from the airport, but I want to see him also and thank him for watching over everything. I saw his moped go by while you were sleeping. He always watches over the place for me when I go away. Want to come with me to meet him? He and his spouse Ben are such great people. I work with them at the school and you will just love them. It is only a few houses down there," she said pointing down the row of boats swaying back and forth.

"No thank you," Stephanie said, feeling her stomach try to turn again just seeing them moving. "I was thinking I might just stay here and take a shower and try to relax some more, that is if you have bathrooms with showers on here and I don't need to get in the ocean water to take one," Steph added dryly, trying to joke with out much luck being funny.

"Well my lady, you just happen to be in luck. We have since stopped showering and bathing in the ocean water months ago. Now we have showers and tubs and even indoor potties now days in all the houseboats, in fact I have two full bathrooms on this boat myself. However; they are a bit smaller than full sized powder rooms in a house per se, but if my big butt fits then yours will I am sure," Susan said, trying to keep the mood light.

Taking Stephanie's hand she showed her around to the bathroom as well as the towel closet, where everything was and how to work the tub, as it was different from land tubs. She gave her a kiss and a hug then she was off.

# CHAPTER 34

"Damn it, a houseboat. I cannot believe it. It didn't even once dawn on me to ask what kind of place she lived in, it is the ocean and I guess it makes perfect sense," Steph said chastising herself. "What do I even really know about this woman? Stop it," she told herself, "you're just cranky. You know you love her and that's all that matters. Go shower and be nice, she kept telling herself."

As she was heading to the bathroom, she walked past the study and stopped dead in her tracks. Trying to get a better look into the room she pushed the door open a little wider with her foot, not sure she was seeing what she knew she was seeing. "Stay calm," she told herself, "just stay calm, it was all before she ever knew you, give her a chance."

She wasn't sure what startled her more, the fact that the whole room was done in pictures of Tiffany and another woman that she didn't know, but felt that she might be the one girl that had died back while they were in college. There was also love letters tacked to the wall as well as other things, or was it the fact that there sitting plain as day on top of the computer screen right in the middle was a little black velvet box with a big diamond ring in it.

The room looked like a room you would see in a movie where someone was obsessed with another person, this

Stephanie thought must be the ring Susan was telling her about that she gave to Tiffany on Christmas morning a long time ago and that Tiffany just threw back at her. Why would she keep it all these years she wondered, it didn't make any sense to keep something around that just hurt you and brought back old bad memories every time you saw it.

As she was pulling the door shut she saw under the edge of the desk a gun laying in a drawer that was half open and a note laying next to it, something about it caught her eye, it was a list of things to do. Number one in bold red marker said "GET OVER TIFFANY IN ANY WAY I CAN!" and then the list went on. Stephanie wondered if she was just a rebound to help Susan get over Tiffany or was the gun her way of doing it? She knew she had to get out of the room or she was going to be sick to her stomach.

All during Stephanie's shower she could not get what she had seen in that room out of her head. After she finished up she decided to go out onto the deck to see if Susan had returned yet.

Susan was sitting over on a corner of the deck reading the newspaper as Stephanie emerged from below.

"Hi baby, I am trying to catch up on the news some. You at least look like you feel better, do you?" Susan wanted to know.

"Sort of," Stephanie answered. "I didn't know if you were back yet or not."

221

"Yes, I have been back for a few minutes. I didn't stay too long just long enough to say hi and see how things went and of course to tell them all about you. They were shocked that I brought someone home as I have never done that before," she said with a smile, "but they can't wait to meet you."

Susan noticed that Steph's mind seemed to be somewhere else, "A penny for your thoughts."

Susan could tell something was bothering Steph and she was sure she had not heard a word that she had just said.

"Susan," Stephanie hesitated before saying, "have you let Tiffany go? I mean really let her go all the way?"

"Stephanie, why would you even ask me that question? I love you and I am with you and I want to be with you. For you to ask me that makes me think you don't trust all that I have said to ..."

Susan stopped in mid sentence, "I think I know why you asked me that. Please remember that we just got here, when I left I thought I was still in love with her and I didn't know you, or else that room would have been take care of. When she moved she left a lot of things behind when we were in college. I know it is silly that I have kept the stuff all these years but, I never let go of the hope at least of her not until I met you and you helped me do that. Also, as for the wall covered in pictures of her, and her and I, I was really into photography in school so that is why that wall is like that, there is even some up of Brittany. I think at one point I was obsessed with Tiffany even to tell you the truth. That has been sometime ago. I have not even gone into that room in a long time other than right before I left to make my to do list as I always do and to get Tiffany's home information in case I would need it. If you had read the list in there you would see that I wanted to get over Tiffany, number one and then the last one was to clean out the study when I returned home. I will take care of it, I promise."

"I did see the pictures as well as the list. I didn't see the last one about cleaning the room out as I only read number one. It bothered me but what bothered me more was the gun laying next to it."

"Oh my God, you didn't think I would have used it did you? I never would have," she reassured Stephanie, "that is not why I have it."

Seeing the disbelieving look on Stephanie's face Susan went on, "Honey I have that gun as a reminder of how bad guns are and it was the only reminder that I have of my brother. It was the only thing I could sneak out of the house with me the night my father kicked me out. I never told you but that is the gun that killed my brother. I promise you that I will tell you all about it later, unless you feel we need to talk about it now?"

"No, later is fine. I feel better now, I was just so worried when I read what it said and then I saw that gun. I even wondered for a minute if I was a rebound to get over her. I now know I am not," she said seeing Susan start to say something as she was shaking her head. "But I don't want to talk about it anymore right now. Let's please just let the subject drop for now anyway, what was then, isn't anymore now, right?" Stephanie asked.

"That's right, it was all in the past," Susan said, relieved.

"Ok then, enough said. I feel better about it all now."

"I will take care of it honey, I promise."

"I said enough Susan, please. There is just too much going on in my head right now. I do not want to complicate things anymore than they are. I think I will go for a walk to clear my head, alone," she added.

Hearing the anger and even a little hurt in Steph's voice Susan let it drop. Feeling dejected and left out of Steph's feelings caused Susan to pout for a while as Stephanie went off to lick her wounds alone.

Susan decided after she got over being upset to clear the room out tonight. Thinking that there was no reason to wait any longer and knowing it hurt Stephanie with it being like it was. She retrieved some boxes and a plastic container she had in her shed to store the items in until she could ask Tiffany if she wanted any of her old stuff back. A couple of hours later she was feeling better, the night air helped remove some of the cobwebs she thought was in her head.

The only thing she decided to keep out was the heavy jacket that she had bought that Christmas long ago, as she had never even used it. She decided she could pack it to go back with her when they went back to either live or visit. Seeing the ring on the computer she decided to put it in the pocket of the jacket until she decided what she wanted to do with it later. She knew she would not give it to Stephanie, as that would be wrong, but she didn't know how to handle that part. She decided to keep the gun out; she would show it to Stephanie when she explained the whole story to her one day.

As Stephanie got back to the boat it was almost dark. She saw Susan going in and out of the boat. She stood back in the shadows and watched as Susan carried some boxes out the door to a little storage shed down below.

As Steph looked around she saw a big trashcan sitting right over from the boat at the edge of the pier, not two feet from the storage room. What Stephanie couldn't figure out was why she wasn't throwing the boxes in there, she knew what was in them. She couldn't figure out also why it was so important to have Susan get rid of the stuff, or why she felt jealous. Telling herself Tiffany was the past and that her and Susan was the future she was able then to get a grip of her thinking.

Stephanie decided to wait until Susan was done before going back. She felt that she might need her space to say good-bye.

"Hey you," Susan said as Stephanie got back up on deck. "I hope you had a nice walk. I meant to tell you before you left that not three blocks down there is the large buoy and it is the marker for the most southern tip of the US. I love walking there at night when there is no tourists around to bother me," she added with a smile. "I made some ice tea. Would you like a glass?"

"Sure," Stephanie said. "It might help combat this smothering heat. So you said I would get use to this heat, right?" as she slapped a big mosquito.

"It took me a little bit," Susan said, "but not too long. How about we go skinny-dipping? I am sure it will help cool you off or make you hot, one of the two?"

"Is there some where around here for that?" Stephanie asked.

"Sure, I know a great place, lets go." She grabbed two big towels as they headed out.

It didn't take them long to get to the spot that Susan knew about. "This is another one of my hiding places to get away from the world. I love to skinny dip and I do it every chance I get."

Susan was out of all her clothing right away, but she had to coax Steph's clothing off of her.

"This feels so weird, a good weird mind you," Stephanie said. "Just this morning I was in a blizzard and now I am going swimming. Ok, so this part I could get use to or maybe even learn to like," Steph added with a smile. "I like being in the water just not on top of it. I have never been skinny dipping though. Are you sure we won't be seen?"

"Well now I made no promises that no one will see us but live a little, that is half the fun in doing it," Susan said with a smile.

"What? Thinking you will get caught?" Stephanie asked.

"Yes," she answered then added, "Last one in has to give the other a back rub," Susan shouted as she ran to the waters edge.

Steph looked around a bit more timidly, seeing no one she ran to the water also.

Susan came up behind her in the water and whispered in her ear, "Since you have never seen the ocean I know you have never made love in the ocean yet," she added." So would this bother you if I was to do this?" she said as she ran her fingertips lightly along Stephanie's neck.

Stephanie shook her head.

"Well then," Susan whispered, "come here baby."

As she reached around Steph's arms she could feel her nipples harden as she brushed them lightly. As she trailed little kisses down Steph's back all the way to her hips she could taste the salt drops on her skin and feel her shiver under her hands.

Susan lead her to the shallow waters edge, as she sat down she pulled Stephanie down with her. She opened her legs so Stephanie sat between them, with her back leaning up against Susan's breast and stomach.

Stephanie cried out when Susan's hands ran the length of her body then came to rest between her legs. As her

227

fingers made little circle movements on Steph's clit, she arched her pelvis upwards so she could feel Susan's fingers pressing into her more.

Susan refused to hurry the rhythm up; she could feel how slippery Stephanie was becoming, even through the salt water. Stephanie arched her hips up and down in unison with Susan's fingers riding the pleasure feelings out; but of a sudden she pushed Susan's hands away.

As she turned around she saw the look in Susan's face as she stood up and pulled her up with her. Leading her to where they lay their towels she spread them out as Susan watched her. When she was done she sat down on her knees and patted the towel next to her. As Susan sat down she leaned over and started kissing her with a hunger they both had. When she could stand it no more she lay Susan back and then she straddled her, putting her hip over Susan's face so she could feel her breath on her pussy.

Susan wrapped her arms around Stephanie to hold her in place as she allowed her tongue to get lost in Steph's salty wetness.

Stephanie undulated her hips against Susan's mouth and tongue, knowing she would not be able to hold out for long like this. She felt Susan's hips arching in rhythm. Stephanie knew she had to taste her also; she wanted them to cum at the same time. Turning around proved hard as Susan was sucking on her clit and didn't want to let it go. Somehow Stephanie managed and as soon as Susan felt

Steph's mouth start sucking and licking at the same time as she shoved two fingers into Susan's pussy, she could hold back no more.

She rode Susan's face and fucked her at the same time with her hand and mouth; they both started bucking together as they both came. Susan took several minutes to catch her breath but she wasn't done. As Stephanie was about to roll over off her she said, "Oh no you don't, I am not done with you yet," she said as she pulled Stephanie's ass back down. She let her tongue start exploring. Within seconds Stephanie was arching up as her body shook and quivered at the complete assaulting her pussy was getting from Susan's mouth. She cried out in pleasure as she came when she felt Susan's tongue slide inside her at the same time Susan's finger slid into her ass.

# CHAPTER 35

"Excuse me, Miss, I am sorry to wake you but I need to get out to use the restroom. Miss, excuse me, please wake up?"

"I'm sorry," Tiffany said as she moved her legs so the woman could get out.

Looking at her watch she knew they still had several more hours in the air before they got there. Standing up to stretch, Tiffany wondered what she was really doing here. She never much liked doing things on her own; she had even surprised herself with wanting to come on this trip at all.

"May I get you some head phones so you can watch the movies?" the flight attendant asked seeing that Tiffany was awake now. Smiling at her, she added with a wink, "When I came around before you were asleep and I didn't want to bother you, as you looked so sweet and cute," Tiffany was sure it was a come on.

"Sure," Tiffany answered dryly without a smile for her in return, meeting someone new was the last thing on her mind right now.

Tiffany tried to lose herself in the movie that was being shown. She loved Meg Ryan but for some reason this time Meg was not holding her attention at all.

"Sorry, I don't mean to bother you again," tapping Tiffany on the shoulder, "but could I please get back in?"

This lady was beginning to bug her already and they had a long flight still to go ahead of them. She sure hoped she wasn't a talker. She just wanted to pretend to watch the movie and get lost in her own self-pity party she was throwing for herself.

"So have you ever been to Australia before?"

"Excuse me?" Tiffany said.

"This is my first trip to Australia and I was just wondering if you had ever been there before," the woman asked again.

"No," Tiffany answered, "this is my first trip there also."

Another few minutes passed before the woman said, "By the way, my name is Cindi. I just hate how close they put these seats to each other, don't you? You cannot get out of them for anything without disrupting the whole row."

"Well, to tell you the truth I had never given it much thought before now, but you're right it would seem. And hello, my name is Tiffany."

Cindi interrupted Tiffany's concentration several more times before she knew it was hopeless with the movie and gave up trying to keep up with it. She was trying not to be rude to this woman, but it was getting harder and harder. She could not see going through the rest of the long flight like this.

The pilot announced that they would be serving dinner soon so she decided to make her break and go wash up as best as she could in the little tiny lavatories on board.

When Tiffany got back to her seat Cindi was waiting on her.

"I didn't want to start eating until you got back," she said. "I thought it might be rude and I have never liked eating alone."

"Thank you, I think," Tiffany said, not knowing what to say at all. Then it seemed like Cindi had decided they knew each other well enough now as she had asked Tiffany to move so she could go to the lavatory. They did exchange names after all, so Tiffany should not have been surprised when she wanted to pick at her food.

"Taste some new things," she said as she offered a fork full of her own food, trying to get Tiffany to sample it in trade to sample some of Tiffany's.

Only then did Tiffany ask her to please back off a bit, she had not come on this trip to meet new people, she was here to get away from people and to be left alone.

Cindi was taken aback by Tiffany's abruptness but not for long. She then decided this woman needed to come out of her funk and she felt she was the woman to do it.

Over the next few hours Tiffany had no other choice but to loosen up as Cindi didn't take hints well. They started talking a bit more and the trip did seemed much shorter.

Just as they were starting to get to know one another, they were told that they would be landing in about thirty minutes.

"I was wondering if you might like to get together while we are here?" Cindi asked. "We could do the touristy things together or dinner or something, since we're both going to be staying in the same city."

Tiffany thought that Cindi was nice and safe enough, and a familiar face in a strange country might be nice after all. They decided to exchange information and hotel numbers as the plane was landing, then they said their good byes with a promise to get together while they were both there.

Tiffany found customs a nightmare and was so glad to be through with all that until she emerged from the airport in Perth, Australia. The rain was coming down in buckets. She had to ask herself again what she was doing here as the sweltering heat and hot rain hit her.

After several frustrating minutes with no luck in getting a taxi, one pulled up to the curb where she stood getting drenched, "Get in," Cindi shouted over the rain.

As Tiffany thankful for a friendly face, got in the cab she said, "Are you sure your driver doesn't mind? I could not get one to stop for anything, they kept honking and yelling something at me, and I don't think it was anything nice either."

"Heck no, why would he get mad? He will get his money's worth I am sure," Cindi answered. "And it is a good thing I had not left yet you would have never gotten a taxi girl, what were you doing anyway?"

"Why what was I doing wrong? What do you mean?" Tiffany asked, taken aback.

"Well dear, in this country they drive on the other side of the road. Everything is turned around, so therefore you were on the wrong curb, they thought you were either waiting on someone or was as dumb as a tack, I'm sure," she added laughing.

Laughing and feeling like a fool herself Tiffany decided to just sit and blush and keep her mouth shut.

"Cute," Cindi said seeing the blush spreading over Tiff's face.

Tiffany pretended to not notice Cindi's leg inch closer to hers in the back of the cab. She was not sure what to make of it, if anything at all even.

The ride to their hotels was long as the rain made it slow going. As the taxi pulled up to Tiffany's hotel first, they both found that they neither one had bothered to get money changed over.

"Oh," Tiffany groaned, "This is just not my day."

"I will take care of this," Cindi said, "as long as you have dinner with me tonight," she added. "I don't know a soul here and it will be nice to have someone to talk to."

"Well I was planning on crashing with room service and a hot bath tonight, but seeing that you rescued me from drowning and also with possible jail for not paying the cabbie you got a deal. How about around 7:00?" she said with a smile.

"Sounds great, 7:00 it is. I look forward to it," Cindi added, "see ya then."

Tiffany was perplexed, she had not gotten any vibes from Cindi, other than a roaming leg and a few quick brushes of her body. She seemed nice enough and she was a doctor, so she felt ok with the dinner, safe at least she told herself.

"Even though she wasn't married as far as Tiffany knew as she didn't wear a ring nor did she talk about a husband or wife for that matter," she said correcting herself. "Well," she reasoned, "she was being insensitive, she just didn't seem gay to her, hell how would I know?" Tiffany chastised herself, "I would not know a lesbian if I tripped over one."

A quick shower and a nap after she got to her room, and she was ready to find something to wear. After looking through her clothing three times she got her best dress out. They had not agreed on what sort of restaurant they would be going to. She decided to try the dress on.

"What am I doing?" she asked her reflection in the mirror. "This isn't a date, it is two new friends having dinner in a huge strange city and a nice causal outfit would work well anywhere they went," she thought.

She went back to the closet and decided on some black slacks, a light blue sweater shirt and some flat shoes. "I'll at least feel comfortable in this," she said to her reflection.

Tiffany was about to call Cindi to let her know she was ready and could meet her downstairs, in the bar, before dinner when she realized that she could not remember her hotel information. She didn't remember where she put the paper with the information on it either.

About that time there was a knock on the door. She found as she approached the door that her hands were shaking, "Calm down," she told herself. "She is just a friend, she knew she was bad at meeting new people but this was ridiculous," she thought as she opened the door.

"Hello, please come on in," Tiffany said as she stepped back. "I am so glad you showed up. We never set where we were to meet and to be honest I lost the information we exchanged already, I should have warned you about that. I am so bad at losing things."

"No worries," Cindi said with a smile. "I'm here now, so let's go do the city, we can stop off at the bar downstairs to have a drink to calm our nerves first," she said seeing Tiffany's hands shaking, "and to also kick off our evening," she added with a smile, "the rain has let up and we both, I think, have a lot of demons to get out tonight."

"I agree," Tiffany said, smiling as they went out the door.

The bar was pretty empty and all the TVs were turned to a soccer match. As they ordered their drinks, they started talking sports with the two men sitting at the bar with them. Both women could not figure out why this country insisted that the game they were half watching on TV was called football, when it was clearly soccer.

The men were half drunk and wanted to argue the fact that Americans were wrong in naming their sports, but was willing to forgive the women's ignorance if they would be willing to have dinner with them tonight.

Tiffany watched in amazement as Cindi said, "Thank you kind sir's," with more manners and politeness than Tiffany would have been able to muster up herself, "but I am afraid we are going to have to beg off tonight as I have thus agreed to have dinner with my very good friend here. I do not want to lead you on, but as it happens to be my womans time of the month I must decline." Seeing the confused look on their faces she added, "I bleed really heavy during my cycle so I am afraid I would be terrible company, you know how PMS'ing women are."

Seeing the disgusted looks on their faces was too much as she had to hide her snickers and smile in Tiffany's shoulder, pretending a big cramp had taken her body over to all most convulsive stages.

The gentlemen assured them that they understood totally and then they bid them a good night, as they headed out the bar quickly, not looking back.

Both ladies were dying laughing as they each knew it was a truly brilliant lie but one that worked most effectively. The bartender came over and said he would be mad for us running his only other two customers out of the bar if it had not been such an awesome lie. It was one of the best he has seen anyone do to fend someone off without any feelings getting hurt at all. He also said he would be telling this story of his two American customers for a long time to come.

It was doing no more than drizzling as they emerged from the bar, so they decided to walk to the restaurant. On the way they had a couple more laughs over the bar escapade.

"That was the best acting I have ever seen," Tiffany said. "I was so wondering how we were going to get out of that one; I think you must have used it before as it was just too convincing," she added with a smile.

"Well you know a girl's got to do what a girl's got to do," she added with a wink. "I go away a lot to conventions and such so most of the time I travel alone. I found in the states that the thing that wards a man off quicker than anything is the first sign of PMS, and they run for the hills. Hell a man is a man, how different could they be in this country? So I knew it would work."

All during dinner Tiffany was trying to figure Cindi out. She didn't think she had ever met anyone quite like her. They found small talk came easy to them. Many drinks later when dinner was over, Tiffany could feel the tension in the air and she didn't think it was just the stranger tensions you get when you just meet someone either. She still wasn't sure what to make of this woman; she had not so much as touched her arm since the cab ride from the airport, and Tiffany didn't know if she wished she would touch her or not.

"So tell me about yourself," Cindi cut into Tiffany thoughts.

"Well," Tiffany began, "where do I start? It's so unbelievable to even me now, it even seems like a lifetime ago. Just two short weeks ago I was getting married to a wonderful guy and I fucked that up all because I didn't love him in that way, so I did what I hope is the right thing and called the wedding off. And now the person I do love that way doesn't love me any more. To top it off, I am here on his and my honeymoon ticket, and if I wasn't plastered I would not be telling you any of this," she added.

"Wow," Cindi said, "that is pretty heavy but not unbelievable. I just never would have guessed that would be your answer."

"Why is that?" Tiffany wanted to know.

"Well to tell you the truth I had you pegged for a lesbian, I guess I should say I'm sorry for assuming, but I think I will say shit, just my luck instead," Cindi added.

Taken aback Tiffany said, "Why would you say that, or assume that I was? Do you think I look like one or what?"

"Well no, it isn't about looks or even labels, but I did notice you have an eye for the ladies. I was watching you as some walked by on the plane as well as here in the restaurant. Also you were so easy to talk with on the plane and I don't get that a lot so I just thought you were. I am sorry; I guess maybe I was just hoping is all."

"Well to tell the truth, ever since the cab ride I have wondered if you were straight or gay myself," Tiffany said, "I guess I have my answer now. I am relieved also as I can be myself and not worry about being judged by you, what ever myself is anyway," she added before seeing Cindi's face, she then wished she could take it back, what ever it was that she said that upset her.

"Ok, first let me make this clear to you. I am not a lesbian and second I would never judge you or anyone else for that matter," Cindi said. "I have a husband and a child, a wonderful little girl at home, that I love very much. I do admit that I was hoping to maybe have my first lesbian experience while I was here but that doesn't make me one."

Tiffany had a twinge of guilt when she heard Cindi say that just because she wanted to try being with a woman didn't make her a lesbian, because she could hear herself all during college saying the same thing.

"I'm sorry. I didn't mean to assume anything. You don't wear a ring so I didn't know you were married," Tiffany said. "And to answer my own question, I am a...one of them," she finished. "That was what all the drama was about back home. I didn't love him like I should have to marry him and I do love her like that but she now doesn't love me. That is why I had to get away."

"Well I think you have had enough drama in your life for a bit, why don't we just have fun and forget all else except this trip being fun, and we can just let what may happen, happen."

"I agree, let's go for it, come on," Tiffany said pulling Cindi to her feet. "I want to live a little."

"I saw a jazz club on the way in, not a block away. If you like jazz that is," she added, "we don't even need to drive. Which is good because I am too tipsy to try to drive. I bet I could get the wrong side of the road part right though," she said with a giggle.

"Well it's good that it's so close as I am so plastered I couldn't drive either, so walk we shall."

"I see the rain has picked back up but I am sure we will not melt, it might even help cool me off," Tiffany added with a smile. "Lets go."

"So you are a little hot are you?" she said with raised eyebrows, "Come on, I'm game. Let's go," Cindi added.

As the night rolled into morning they both were about ready to call it a night, the bars here never closed and they were still working on the USA time frame.

Cindi was on the dance floor doing a shag dance when she saw Tiffany heading to the ladies room. She didn't like the way some of the men were watching her, and she knew Tiffany was wasted even more than she herself was. She was afraid for her to go alone so she excused herself from the dance and took off after her, as Cindi got in the bathroom door Tiffany was leaning over the sink washing her face with cold water. Seeing Cindi come in the door she smiled at her, surprised that she came in.

"Hi," Tiffany said. "I thought you were dancing. I started having hot flashes from all the drinks I think so I wanted to wash my face."

"I saw some of the crude men that wouldn't leave you alone before watching you walk this way and it is so dark and out of the way back here I didn't want you in here alone," Cindi offered as she handed Tiffany some paper towels to dry off with.

"Thank you," she said as she took the towels. "For these," she said looking at the towels, "and for being here with me tonight. I thought all I wanted was to be alone but I can tell it wasn't what I needed." She could feel the tears welling up and she tried to hide them but Cindi saw.

"Come here," she said as she took Tiffany into her arms. She let her cry for a bit, "Ok now, dry it up and wash your face. This trip isn't about anyone back home, remember this is our time?" she added with a smile.

After a few sniffles more and a good blowing of her nose, Tiffany felt a little better. She knew what Cindi had said was right, and she didn't intend to come all the way to another country to sit and cry the whole time about Susan. She was not going to feel sorry for herself or let Cindi feel sorry for her either.

"Come on," Tiffany said, grabbing her hand, "let's do one more shot and head back, ok?"

Cindi didn't answer; she just leaned against the sink looking at Tiffany. She had Tiffany's hand in hers already so she gently pulled Tiffany to her.

"What are you doing?" she whispered as she came to a stop with her breast resting against Cindi's.

"This," Cindi whispered as she leaned forward and brushed her lips softly against Tiffany's, she could feel her heart beating in her chest. This was the first time she had ever kissed a woman and she liked the feel of the soft lips against hers. She let their kissing grow deeper; she tested the water by letting her tongue slightly part Tiffany's lips. Feeling Tiffany responding drove her tongue deeper still. She could feel the desire growing in her as she slowly moved her hands up along side Tiffany's breasts and gently cupped one of them in her hand. She could feel how soft it was even through the fabric of Tiffany's sweater.

"Are you sure you want to do this?" Tiffany managed to get out through Cindi's tongue and mouth.

Cindi moaned her answer as her other hand moved up under Tiffany's shirt. As her fingers touched Tiffany's naked breast for the first time, she felt twinges deep in her pussy that she had not felt before, even with her husband.

Tiffany was unsure as to how much Cindi would allow her to do or even how much she would want her to do, so she just ran her hands over her back and arms, returning the kisses with the same want and passion. She knew Cindi could tell she wanted her; there would be no mistaking that. She would just let her have the lead.

After several minutes of kissing and fondling as if they were schoolgirls Cindi pulled back saying, "I am a little unsure as to how far you are willing to go with me. I know you're drunk and I do not want to do anything you will regret when we sober up."

"I'll have regrets if you stop here," Tiffany said as she unbuttoned her slacks for Cindi.

Getting the message loud and clear Cindi raised Tiffany's shirt up so she could see if her nipples felt as good in her mouth as they had in her hands. As she sucked on her nipple rough and hard Tiffany cried out in a pleasure pain causing Cindi to pull back a little bit.

"No," Tiffany said. "Don't stop. It didn't hurt in a bad way. I liked it," she said as she pulled Cindi's head back onto her breast. Tiffany was now leaning up against the sink holding on to the edge now with her head laid back. "Cindi, she could tell, liked nipples," she thought with a smile.

Tiffany felt herself getting very wet. As all her muscles were jerking and contracting she wanted so badly to reach down into her pants and stroke herself but she wanted Cindi to do that also and she didn't want to send the wrong message to her. She was afraid she would think I didn't want her to do it herself she though.

Cindi, as if reading her mind, stood up and replaced her mouth with one of her hands. As her fingers were squeezing her nipple hard her other hand made its way to the top of her pants. She slowly unzipped them and let them fall off her hips a little bit. She could tell Tiffany was wearing no underwear and this made her hotter. She let her fingers massage on their way to her lips, using her fingers she slowly pulled them apart, she could tell by how wet Tiffany was that she was enjoying herself.

As she let her finger slowly touch her clit, Tiffany's body jerked. Cindi wanted to make Tiffany wait, she was sure that she was the type of girl that never had to wait for anything in her life. So she lightly rubbed and tapped and pulled everything but her clit. With every touch Tiffany was jerking and pleading for release. Cindi wasn't about to give in just yet, with this woman she was going to be everything she wasn't at home; she was going to be in control and not be timid at all.

"Please baby, I can't stand this," Tiffany begged, "I want to feel your fingers in me and I want to ride your hand. You have got me so wet and hot, don't do this to me."

Cindi was paying no attention to her words at all, her mouth had found the other breast and she was punishing it good. She knew her teasing fingers were driving Tiffany mad.

Tiffany decided she could stand no more so she started to reach her hand into her pants when Cindi stopped her by grabbing her hand and pinning it to her side. Standing up, her mouth captured Tiffany's and muffled her cries when Cindi rammed her hand into Tiffany all at once. She was nice and wet so her hand slid in easily from all Tiffany's juices covering it. As she was fucking her hard, Tiffany didn't notice the bathroom door open and two ladies walk in. Cindi caught sight of them in the mirror; she saw the expression on their faces and knew they would not send anyone in. They watched her keep fucking Tiffany for a few minutes, then turned and left, giving them their privacy.

"Fuck, I'm cumming!" Tiffany said as she grabbed hold of Cindi's arm and rode her hand hard. At one point Cindi was afraid that they were being too rough, she knew she would be sore tomorrow.

When Tiffany let loose of her grip, she leaned back with her back against the mirror and her eyes closed. Cindi leaned over and kissed her mouth gently this time.

"This is going to be a wonderful trip," she whispered to Tiffany.

They walked out of the bathroom after getting themselves fixed up and the two ladies were standing by the door. "All done," Cindi said with a wink, recognizing them. "Thanks," she whispered to one of them.

"I hope they didn't hear us," Tiffany said a bit worried, looking back over her shoulder at the two women watching them, with big smiles on their faces.

246

Knowing that they were the two that had came in on them and also knowing they had stood and watched for them to keep others out, Cindi said with a smile, "I hope they did."

.............................................................

...........

"God, I have not had a hang over like this in a long time," Tiffany said, holding her head in her hands, "not since college."

"Dang, turn out the lights," Cindi said.

"Get up," Tiffany told her. "That's not lights, that's the sun. Dang, it's almost 3:00 in the afternoon."

"I can't even remember most of last night, and oh, my head," Cindi added. "I remember I helped you in here and I just wanted to shut my eyes for a minute, that's it, I remember no more. I think I passed out along with you."

"I see we both passed out in all our clothing," Tiffany added as she threw the covers back to the muddy mess they had made from being soaked from the rain. Laughing, they both groaned at the same time.

"No jokes, my head cannot take it," Cindi said. "I knew I drank a lot but I didn't know it was that much. I've got to go shower and clean up. I think I am going to change hotels if you don't mind, that is if they have a room available," she added.

"Why don't you?" Tiff started, "Never mind," she then said.

"No, go on, finish it. What is it that you were going to say?" Cindi wanted to know.

"Well I was just going to say you could stay here with me in my room, with no strings attached, of course really no strings at all. I am here to get over, not into another relationship and I think it would be nice to have a friend to hang around with, we both want to see the country a bit so when we get the rental we can go together, what do you think?"

After thinking about it for a minute Cindi finally said, "Sure, I don't see why not, I think that will be ok. If you're sure you do not mind."

"Hey," Tiffany said, "just so you know. I wasn't too drunk that I don't remember last night. I do not regret any of it," she added with a smile, "and thank you."

"You don't need to thank me," Cindi said. "I think you could tell I was enjoying it myself also, or at least I hope you could."

"I didn't know how much or how far you would let me go so I gave you all the control," Tiffany said, trying not to blush as she remembered more of last night.

"As for last night, it went as far as I wanted it to go. I have this warped way of thinking that as long as I don't let anyone do me; I'm not cheating on my husband. Then the other part of my brain tells me as long as I am with a woman it isn't cheating either, as I have already talked it over with my husband. It is with his blessing that I explore this side of me. So we will just play it by ear."

"I think your way of thinking about it is different," Tiffany said. "But that doesn't mean it is good or bad way, just different," she said, looking into Cindi's eyes.

"I will tell you, when you are so close to me, I don't know if I can control myself," she said as she ran her fingers down Tiffany's cheek and over her shoulders.

Tiffany decided to go shower first, she left the door open so they could talk but she was not aware of Cindi watching her shower through the glass tub doors. She kept watching as she got out of the tub and toweled off.

"I am going to go shower now and think about what we were talking about some more now that I have a clear head," Cindi said as Tiffany came out of the bathroom in her bathrobe. "And one more thing about what you said about giving me power," Cindi said as she turned around a looked at Tiffany on her way to the bathroom. I don't know that you gave me the control," Cindi said with a smile. "I think I pretty much took it and a lot more from you last night," she added with a twinkle in her eye.

Now Tiffany was really blushing as Cindi walked back to where she sat on the bed; she then leaned forward and kissed her.

Cindi smiled, "I don't regret it either. As a matter of fact I was really turned on, you didn't get the chance to feel but I was as soaked as you, if not worse. I hope we can explore that side of our new friendship further. I was wondering if you would remember it or not so I wasn't going to bring it up just in case. Besides, who says friends can't have fun also?" she added a wink to make her point.

"I think I will agree with you on that one about friends," Tiffany said, as the blush spread across her cheeks at an alarming rate.

Cindi took her turn in the bathroom trying to get herself straightened up a little bit, and she left the door open also but not so they could talk. She did it so that Tiffany could watch her shower, she planned on giving her a show.

Tiffany passed by the bathroom to get her clothing out of the closet she saw Cindi getting into the shower, she almost felt embarrassed to stand there and watch as she backed away from the door a little bit. When she had backed up against the closet door she stopped and opened it stepping half way in pretending to look for something to wear as she watched Cindi.

Cindi had taken the soap and lathered up the washcloth, she then started slowly washing her right leg, she could see out of the corner of her eye that she had her desired audience watching from outside the bathroom. As she washed her other leg she then moved up her body, lathering herself up good. Missing certain parts that she wanted to save for later. Putting her washcloth down, she grabbed the soap and lifted one leg up on the side of the tub. She got the razor and started shaving her leg slowly trying to rub her upper leg as sensual as she could as she worked the razor.

She could tell it was working as she could see Tiffany switching her weight from one foot to the other.

Tiffany was finding watching Cindi when she didn't know she was being watched very exciting. And the thought that Cindi might catch her was even more intriguing to her. She didn't know that someone shaving their body could be so stimulating.

She stood up and rinsed all the soap off her body. She then soaped up again, this time using nothing but her hands as she slowly ran her hands over her body, arching just a bit as she rubbed.

When her hand slipped over her breast and nipples she rolled her head back just a bit, she then let one of her hands run down her body, trailing soap as she went. As she let her hand slip between her legs, she started slowly rubbing the soap back and forth.

She could still see Tiffany watching her as she stood half in the closet, she could see that her robe had fallen half open.  When she grabbed the showerhead she slowly let the water run down her;  she moved the showerhead down her body as she opened her legs and let it pulsate on her clit for a minute causing her body to jerk slightly but enough for Tiffany to see it.

She knew she was working Tiffany into a frenzy as well as herself, she then decided it was enough of a show unless she was going to go all the way.

Cindi replaced the showerhead to the top of the shower. Tiffany knew she was getting ready to get out of the tub, so she hurried to the bed forgetting her clothing. Her face was hot and flushed, and she knew she was very wet.

Tiffany sat and thought about Cindi in the shower and about last night at the club, mainly about the time they spent in the bathroom together. She didn't know why but she felt a little guilty this morning about it. She knew that Susan was out of her life for good and that she had moved on, but this didn't stop Tiff's guilt.

Interrupting Tiffany's thoughts, Cindi walked out of the shower with nothing on but a robe. "I gave it some more thought," she said with a sly smile.

Tiffany was sitting on the bed trying to look innocent as Cindi walked over to her and sat down really close beside her, allowing her legs to open slightly so it rubbed against Tiffany's.

"God I want to kiss you; very badly I might add," Tiffany whispered. "May I?"

"Please do," Cindi said as she let her tongue slip out slightly, parting her lips as she ran her tongue over them, Tiffany watched her every action.

Tiffany could stand no more; she leaned over and kissed Cindi leaving a trail of kisses along her jaw line and down to the little opening on the front of Cindi's robe.

"May I?" Tiffany asked in a husky whisper. Not waiting for an answer, she moved the robe back exposing a breast. Tiffany felt really anxious as she was pretty new to all this. What she did know was long ago forgotten and that wasn't much, years ago. As Cindi started squirming under Tiffany's mouth, she felt more confident as she was trailing little circles around each of Cindi's nipples.

Tiffany was not in the mood for foreplay, watching Cindi in the shower had taken her to the brink just from watching. She wanted to taste Cindi, and she wanted it now. She gently took one of Cindi's nipples between her teeth and pulled it a little bit. She then looked into Cindi's eyes as she pushed her legs apart to kneel on the floor between them.

Cindi half sat up on her arms behind her. Tiffany stopped kissing her stomach thinking she wanted her to stop.

Cindi told her in a slight whisper not to stop; she only wanted to watch her. This turned Tiffany on even more; she spread Cindi's lips open with her fingers and moved her face down to eye level with Cindi's clit. Instead of using her tongue as Cindi expected her to do she blew on it then slowly darted her tongue in and out on it.

"Damn that feels good," Cindi remarked, rolling her head back a little, "don't you dare stop."

Tiffany could hold back no more as she started sucking and biting on Cindi's clit. Letting her tongue flick Cindi's clit cause Cindi to move and arch. She spent some time on her clit until she felt Cindi jerk with every lick not wanting her to cum yet before she had a chance to let her tongue slide into her pussy, and she was far from done with her yet.

Spreading her legs as wide as she could get them, she wanted her tongue as far into Cindi as she could get it to go. Tiffany now knew what a woman tasted like. She now knew what she had been missing by not giving it a try. Being with a woman very much turned her on. Her own pussy got very wet at the taste of Cindi's.

"Damn," Cindi said. "I have dreamed of this. Never once did it ever feel like this," she said as she reached down and pulled her lips open even more for Tiff, she wanted to be as exposed to her as she could.

Tiffany was not about to stop her assault on Cindi's pussy. She wanted to make her cum, and she wanted to hear a woman cry out from what she was doing to them with her mouth and hands. She never told Cindi but this was her first time ever going down on a woman. All the time she was with Susan, Susan was the giver and she the receiver; she could never make herself do that to another woman.

She didn't have to wait long to hear Cindi cry out her name. As her hands were on Cindi's breast and her mouth was all over her pussy suddenly Cindi cried out. "Oh Tiffany, hold on baby I am there, I'm there, oh God I am there!"

254

With that Cindi grew rock still but Tiffany continued to suck and lick, she was not letting up for one minute. Cindi then started rocking back and forth and when her body grew still she reached down and grabbed Tiffany's head and hair to hold her still. Tiffany knew she was done when every flicker of her tongue sent Cindi into fits of giggles.

Looking up at Cindi with a huge smile on her face Tiffany said, "Fuck yeah I'm a lesbian and I like it!" This was the first time she could even say the words without stuttering while she was trying to say them.

Cindi just smiled and giggled at her, she knew this was some sort of breakthrough for Tiffany.

# CHAPTER 36

After making love in the water and then on the sand they dressed and walked hand in hand on the beach for a while. Sunrise wasn't far off, and they both decided they would sit on the end of the pier and watch it together.

"Guess what?" Susan said out of the blue.

"Well give me a hint," Stephanie answered.

"While you were gone for your walk last night, I took care of the study. It didn't take me that long to get it all cleared out."

Stephanie thought for a minute before saying anything, "You didn't need to Susan. I had no right to even wonder about it, I love and trust you, and I knew when you were ready you would do what you felt was right."

"Well I was ready, and you had every right to wonder and ask about it. I figured why wait, just throw it all away and then it would be all over and done with," Susan added with a smile.

"So you threw it all away?" Stephanie asked.

"Yes I did, (sort of)," she added quietly, knowing Stephanie couldn't hear it. Then she went on to say, "I had no need for any of it anymore, now kiss me you fool," Susan said.

Kissing her Steph thought, "Yes, I just might be a fool after all. Or even still, she just might be a fool for lying to me."

"You're pretty quiet this morning," Susan said. "Anything you want to talk about?"

"I was just thinking back to something you said to me last evening after my shower."

"What was that?" Susan asked.

"Well, you said that when you left you were in love with her and that was only two short weeks ago and now I'm here with you and you say you're in love with me. It just makes me feel like this might not be all that real between us to you, since it was so quick. I am starting to feel even more as if I am a replacement as I said before."

"Now don't be silly," Susan said, casually, not taking what Stephanie was saying seriously as they had talked about it already yesterday, and she felt like she had reassured her enough. "You're no replacement for anything or anyone as I all ready told you. I just don't think love knew it was too soon after before it took over my heart again with you. With her I was holding on to a ghost of the past, the long ago past even, not the now. With you it is the here and now."

"What if love didn't know you was done with your feelings for her either?" Stephanie said more perplexed than before.

"Honey, it is alright and we will be alright. Please just trust me. I had to let Tiffany go many years ago. True my heart still held out hope but my head didn't, it knew all along."

"We'll see," was all she felt she could say.

As the sun came up over the water Susan could hear Steph's intake of breath. Neither one said anything as they both sat side-by-side watching, lost in its beauty.

"The sunrises here are very beautiful I must admit," Stephanie said. "They're so different from the ones back home. When you watch the sun come up over the flat look of the water you appreciate how pretty it is. When it comes up over the jagged rocks of the mountains, it is nice also but just in a different way."

They stood up to head towards the boat. "As I was watching the sun come up, I was also thinking I need to say something to you. I don't want you to get upset, but I would like to check into a hotel today. I know me and I know I cannot sleep on the boat. I will stay nauseous the whole trip if I try and stay on board. I don't think you want me sick the whole trip, because I know I can be hateful when I am sick," she added with a smile.

Feeling let down Susan cut in, "But you didn't even give it a chance Stephanie. Could you stay just one night, just for me? I want to share my home with you and I..." deciding not to finish what she was going to say she added, "You didn't even spend one night on the boat and if you would just wait and see I know you would love it like I do." Relishing what Stephanie had said Susan added," Of course I don't want you sick the whole time, and I hope this turns out to be more than just a trip."

"I don't want to talk about it, I am going to find a nice hotel or a cottage that doesn't sway back and forth for the rest of my stay. You are more than welcome to join me. I would really like it if you did, but right now I just cannot take the boat. I get sick to my stomach even thinking about it. Maybe the next time if the waters are not so choppy," she added.

"I wouldn't mind so bad," Susan said, "if I didn't just love the houseboat so much. I just wanted you to love it also, make it our place." Seeing the look that Stephanie had on her face Susan added, "Ok, let's get a cottage. I know where there are some nice ones to rent by the night; I'm not big on hotels. Promise me you will think about giving it another try in a few days after you are feeling better."

Stephanie didn't answer Susan right away. "There is something else bothering you isn't there? You seem so distant right now, that's why I am asking you."

"Yes there is," Stephanie said, "but I do not feel I can talk about it right now. I need time to work it out in my head first then we can talk," she added. "I always need time to process things, I have always been that way I guess it is the writer in me. So please just bare with me a little."

"As you wish," Susan said, standing up. "Come on," she said, holding her hand out to Stephanie. "Let me help you up." Deciding yesterday was a bad enough day. She wasn't going to let today go the same way; she decided she was going to comply with Stephanie's wishes without a fight.

As they walked back to the boat in silence Susan wondered if Stephanie could have seen her taking the boxes to the shed or maybe she hates it here that much. As the nagging thought came to mind that she just might not want her anymore she quickly put it out of her head.

"Nah," she reasoned to herself, "She couldn't have seen and she knew she didn't really lie to Stephanie, but she did feel guilty for stretching the truth way out of shape. Why didn't I just tell her the whole truth? It wasn't a big deal. I am such an idiot." Another thought that crossed her mind was why she felt the need to keep the items in the first place.

"Damn it," she muttered out loud.

# CHAPTER 37

Tiffany and Cindi both tried to tidy themselves up before going downstairs to deal with the front desk. They giggled like schoolgirls all the way downstairs.

They were surprised that it took no more than twenty minutes to square the front desk away. Both of them had to giggle a time or two in the elevator on the way back to the room over the funny looks they received when they told the gentleman at the front desk that they were going to room together. After he pointed out that there was only one bed in the room and that a roll away would cost even more, and that was if they even had one not in use.

That was not near as funny as the sounds he made and the rolling of his eyes as they both said never mind to the roll away, as they didn't need it because they intended to be sharing the same bed.

They were still laughing hard about it when they got to Tiffany's room, so hard in fact, that she found it hard to get her key to work without Cindi's help. After the fits of laughter had subsided Tiffany asked, "Hey, I have a great idea. How about an afternoon swim? My headache has all but gone away, and I think a dip would be refreshing."

"Sounds great," Cindi said, "I have not been swimming since last summer. We have a pool back home, but it isn't heated so no winter swimming at all, unless you're a polar bear," she added with a giggle.

"First I do need to go to my hotel first, to check out and pack all my things back up, want to help?"

"Nah," Tiffany answered, "I need to make some phone calls. I'll be here when you get back though," she added, "waiting on you."

"See ya then. It should take me no more than an hour," Cindi said as she headed out the door.

"Hey," Tiffany called out, "on second thought hold the elevator for me. I changed my mind; I'll go and help you if you still want me to? If you are only going to take an hour or so it will give me plenty of time as it is 5:00 a.m. in the states. I should wait a couple of hours to call home or at least until I know they have woke up," she added with a smile. "Just let me grab my sweater and I'll be right with you."

"Great," Cindi said as Tiffany hurried to the elevator. Once inside the elevator Tiff reached for Cindi's hand and leaned over and gave her a very passionate kiss. She then gave herself a little smile. She felt content for the time in a long time.

As they emerged from Tiff's hotel, still holding hands, they decided to walk to the other hotel. Cindi had said it wasn't that far away, and it was a lovely day, other than a little chill in the air. Tiffany felt alive, for the first time in a long time. It even felt like her skin was alive, holding Cindi's hand. "You know, I believe being here was just what I needed to make a new start."

Cindi just smiled at her and squeezed her hand.

Tiffany knew what they were building was nothing more than a special friendship, and it would go no further than this country. While here, she was going to bask in it, and she was not going to let herself get attached either.

"Who knows?" Cindi said cutting into her thoughts as if she could read them again. "You and I may need to meet up at different times a year for little get together," she added with a smile. "I go to conventions all over many times a year. Most of the time I am always alone. I think it would be great fun to have you there with me at some of them," she said. As she gave Tiff's hand a squeeze she leaned over and kissed her right there out on the sidewalk.

"Oh, great idea. I would like that. I always have hated good-byes. We can just do the bye until next time we meet thing. We can have the kind of seeing one another on a causal basis from time to time at least for some sight seeing and good sex and not always in that order, kind of relationship," Tiffany added, raising her eyebrows, and with that they both laughed.

Even though she felt a slight urge to let lose of Cindi's hand while they were out in public she didn't. She knew she had to get over it. She had already admitted she was a lesbian to herself and out loud to someone that now probably thought she was a fruit for saying it, and that was the hardest thing for her to do. She could deal with this part of it also. "One step at a time," she reminded herself, "one step at a time."

"I can feel you're not comfortable with us holding hands," Cindi cut into Tiffany's thoughts once again. "Would you like for me to let go? I do understand."

"I'm sorry," Tiffany said, "and no I don't want that, it is so uncanny how you can read my thoughts. You've got to remember; in some ways this is all new to me also. You know what? I am not going to let it get the better of me," she finally answered as she grabbed Cindi's arm and pulled her closer.

They were walking slow and talking as they went and they had gotten no more than twenty or thirty feet from Tiffany's hotel entrance doors when a cab pulled up.

"You lassies want me to pack you to where you're going?" he asked, yelling out the window.

"Oh no. But thank you though," Tiffany said with a giggle at the name he called them.

Cindi added to make their point, "It is way too pretty out here today to ride, and we want to be outside as much as we can, so I think we are just going to walk."

"Suit yourselves. I hope you lassies have a nice day," he said as he tipped his cap towards them, and drove away.

"I have got to call mother later today," she said to Cindi. "I promised her I would call her when I got here and got settled in. You may need to remind me later though dear," Tiffany said.

For some reason she was having trouble thinking of anything back in the states while here with Cindi, she thought to herself feeling happy the first time in a long time.

Neither of them saw the four thugs standing in the alleyway as they passed by them. Tiffany felt the first blow to the back of her head as they jumped out at them. She had caught a glimpse of them out of the corner of her eye when they moved out of the shadows towards them. She tried to turn around as she started screaming for them to get away and leave them alone. That was when she felt the second blow to the head that took her to the ground, landing hard on her stomach.

"Don't fight us," one of them spat out, "and we may let you live!"

He grabbed her legs to roll her over, and as he did she managed to kick him in the groin, sending him to the ground also. That just seemed to make them angrier. One of them grabbed the lead pipe and started hitting Tiffany with it as Cindi screamed.

They were holding her back, and she could do nothing to help Tiffany at all. They grabbed hold of her and forced her to watch, Cindi felt helpless.

Tiffany lay there half conscious while they kept beating her. All she could move was her eyes; the rest of her body would no longer move. She could hear them cursing nasty names at them, and she could tell they were angry with them being together. Three of them began kicking and spitting on her, and she could not make her mind understand why they were doing this to them. It was in the middle of the day, and Tiffany knew they were not far from the hotel, what she could not work out was why no one was helping them. After one of them kicked her in the face she could not make her eyes open anymore. They were swollen shut already; she was trying to open them to see if she could see where Cindi was. It proved to be too much for her. The last thing she remembered was feeling something warm running over her face and a bone stabbing pain run through her as something hit her or someone kicked her lower back, she then passed out.

They were holding Cindi back making her watch everything as they beat Tiffany until she passed out in the middle of the sidewalk. She also had to watch as one of them pissed on Tiff's face. His urine mixed with her blood and it ran down and over her face.

Every time Cindi would scream or try to turn away and not watch anymore, the guy holding her would laugh and then spit on her, jerking her arms even tighter behind her.

"We're going to teach you both a lesson," one of the nasty guys with no teeth said. He grabbed Tiffany by the hair dragging her into the alley. Cindi was relieved that Tiffany had since passed out so she didn't have to feel any more of the pain. Cindi could tell she was still breathing, but it was very labored, and she was worried about her.

She heard one of the guys tell the other one to stand watch until his turn. She saw him bring a big knife out; she thought he was going to cut either her or Tiffany, but he used it to cut Tiffany's clothing off of her instead. They forced her to watch as they one by one brutally raped Tiffany's limp body. They threw her around as if she was a rag doll. Cindi knew that Tiffany was still alive and could still feel some of what they were doing to her; she would cry out from time to time in pain as they would move her a certain way.

After they were done with Tiffany they threw her behind a huge garbage bin as if she wasn't even human then they all turned on her. She was crying and begging them to please leave her alone and not to hurt her.

"We hate fags," one of them spat at her, "we're going to teach you what a man feels like," he said as he grabbed her shirt and tore it off of her.

"I'm not gay," Cindi pleaded. "I have a husband and a baby girl," she cried, trying to make them understand. She was in shock from seeing what they did to Tiffany and didn't realize it. Somewhere in the back of her head she thought they would not get out of this alive.

Trying to make them understand, didn't help they didn't care. They grabbed hold of her pants and cut them off, and they threw her to the ground onto her back. She tried to crawl backwards on her hands, but they hit her in the stomach. She still had her underwear on as she felt a hand grab hold of her panties and jerk them off her. She tried not to scream, she didn't want to make them any madder. One of them took hold of her arm and flipped her over as one of the other men grabbed her bra and cut it off.

They each took turns raping her anally. She tried not to black out or cry out too much. She thought they might just rape her and leave her alone as they had not beaten her yet.

They were each taking their turns at assaulting her when one of them got the bright idea to shove his penis in her mouth, while the other one fucked her from behind. When he shoved his penis in she gagged and bit down on him from the reflex. She didn't mean to but he screamed and cursed at her, took his lead pipe and smashed her in the mouth and nose.

She felt blood squirt out everywhere. The men raping her became angry again and got really rough. She could feel herself ripping and tearing, and she could feel hands yanking at her breast and other hands pushed and pulled her body everywhere else. She felt them shove something inside her way too deep, while another one was still raping her. She tried to focus on her daughter back home as she felt herself slipping into the darkness. She could only see Tiffany's legs sticking out from behind the trash bin as she closed her eyes; she knew she was blacking out as they all started beating on her. She saw the guy that she had bit with the knife, and she also saw him start stabbing her over and over again in the neck, head and chest.

She felt relieved that she could not feel any pain from the blade; she could see blood squirting everywhere and then she saw nothing but black when one of them started kicking her in the head.

When the men were satisfied that they had taught both of them a lesson they would never forget, they straightened their clothing up and wiped the blood from the blade of the knife off on Cindi's skin.

One of the guys said his buzz was wearing off, and he was all out of crystal meth and needed another bloody hit, badly.

After rummaging though Cindi and Tiffany's discarded clothing he found some money that Cindi had with her. "Look what I found," he said. "Lets go get some crystal and have us a little party," holding up the money for his buddies to see.

# CHAPTER 38

Susan felt so guilty all day over the little white lie she had told that she knew she had to do something to make it up to Stephanie.

"Andrew? Hi, this is Susan. I need to set up an appointment to look at some houses to rent just for a short time. Yes, this evening will be fine," she said, "thank you, see you then."

As Stephanie came into the room Susan startled her. "Hey honey, I have a surprise for you. I have made us an appointment to go house hunting this evening."

"You did what?" Stephanie said with plenty of anger in her voice, "why ever would you do that? We have not talked about staying here, hell, we have not talked much at all."

Susan was in tears, "I'm sorry I just thought you said you wanted a house on land. You hate it here on the boat, so I thought I would help us find a place just for a few days. I told him it was just for a short time," she said through her tears, "and... and... and..." she tried to keep going as sobs racked her body.

"Oh honey, I'm sorry, I didn't mean to be so mean, I didn't know you were talking about short term, and I guess I just was feeling a little rushed. Come on and lets try this again. Anyway, as I was sitting out on deck I thought of a plan that might work even better," she said with a smile.

Susan stopped crying and sat there sniffling for a few minutes waiting for her to go on.

"Tell you what," Stephanie began, "let's go away for a few days, away from all this. I have a great place in mind. I know we just got here, but I think we got off to a bad start and we just need something fresh. We can then talk, it has just been so stressful."

After thinking about it for a minute, Susan decided that was a wonderful idea, "I think that is great. Let me make all the plans to make it up to you and I..."

"No way," Stephanie cut in, "no telling where we will end up staying or on what," she added with a smile. "Anyway like I said I have something in mind. I will take care of everything, you just go pack."

Susan called Andrew and cancelled the house hunting appointment. She told him to stay on stand by, that she may need him again soon and to keep a look out for some places for her, she would be in touch with him in a week or so. After thanking him, she hung up and went to pack.

Susan knew she had a while still yet before the new school year started but decided to call Ms. Ellen anyway to let her know she would need to be taken off the roster as of right now, but if it changed she would let her know.

"I am sorry that you may not be coming back to join us," Ms. Ellen said, "I hope everything is ok, is there anything wrong?"

"No Ms. Ellen, everything is fine," Susan said, "I just do not know what I will be doing this coming school year, and I didn't want to wait until the last minute to let you know if I could not make it."

"Well if you change your mind please do let me know dear. It isn't for a few more weeks, so take some time to think about it."

She promised her she would give it some thought because she missed the kids already as she did every break they had. "My plans are just all up in air right now, but I will give it some more thought," then she added, "I will let you go now."

Hearing the sadness in her voice all Ms. Ellen said was, "Keep your chin up, and it will all work out. Bye dear"

Stephanie made Susan go for a walk while she made the arrangements and got the rental car. She wanted it to be a total surprise.

When Susan came back to the boat the rental car was there, and Stephanie had it packed with their things and ready to go. All that was left for Susan to do was lock the boat up tight and climb into the car. She felt sadness as she loved her boat, and they had just gotten there, but she knew she had to do it for them.

"Come on, you've got to tell me where we're going, or at least how long it is going to take for us to get there."

Susan pouted as Stephanie drove on, paying no attention to her.

"Stephanie come on now, tell me," Susan pleaded, "I know we are going north," she teased, "since going south we would be swimming with the fishes by now."

"I know you don't really want to know before we get there now do you?" Stephanie said laughing, "but even if you do, I'm not going to tell you, just lay back and rest. It's still several more hours before we get there."

As Susan laid back she was feeling a bit light headed again, so she decided to try and get some sleep to see if that would help, she ended up sleeping during the rest of the drive. She awoke only once for a few minutes during the trip when Stephanie pulled into the gas station to fill up.

Stephanie spent much of the drive doing a lot of soul searching and thinking about everything, and she decided to let all that had happened go and start fresh. "Nothing was worth losing this woman over," she thought, "not even a misunderstanding or a little white lie," the little voice in the back of her head kept saying. "Shake it off," Stephanie said to herself as she drove the rest of the way with a smile on her face.

"What is it with you and the great outdoors?" Susan asked as she woke up when they pulled into the driveway of a lovely little cabin right next to a large creek, and as far as Susan could tell it was in the middle of nowhere.

"You're not disappointed too much are you?" Stephanie wanted to know. "I was sure you would love it."

"Of course I am not disappointed, I am pleasantly surprised even. Where are we anyway?" Susan wanted to know.

"Georgia," Stephanie answered, "I called a friend of mine that owns this cabin. I have always wanted to visit here but never seemed to make the effort, and now, I thought was the perfect time with you next to me. I used to hear her talk about this place when we were in college. I thought it would be ideal to come here to get away and write, but I am glad I saved my first visit here so I could share it with you."

Feeling honored and even guiltier now more than before Susan said, "Stephanie I need to tell you something. This place is wonderful, and I am glad we are sharing it together, but I have felt bad all day about a little fib I told you on the dock when we were watching the sunrise. I am so sorry about it. I didn't mean to stretch the truth and there is no excuse for it. I don't know why I even did. I do hope you will forgive me."

"Shhh," Stephanie cut in, "it's ok, let's leave all that behind us now, believe it or not I understand. I knew about it and I was hoping you would tell me. Now you have and it's over and done with. Ok?"

"Will you please forgive me? I Just need to talk to you about it is all, until I know you have forgiven me. I am just so sorry and...ok, you're right. It's all over and done with, lets move on," Susan added seeing the look on Steph's face.

274

"Now first things first, I have got to pee and you need to take a nap. You drove the whole way here and this seems to be a trend for us," she added with a smile. "I know you have got to be tired."

"I am a little tired," Stephanie, agreed, "maybe a short nap would do me some good. I sort of have a little headache anyway."

As they walked into the house they could tell no one had been there in a long time. They acted like children as they explored the place.

Seeing there was nothing at all in the kitchen that even resembled food, Susan offered to go for a drive and get them some supplies while Stephanie rested.

"I will not be too long," she promised. "And I would love to get out and drive anyway in all this wildlife while it is still light enough to see all I can see," she added with a smile. "I am not big on driving, but I think I will like it here; the trees are huge here and they're everywhere."

"Why don't you just wait until I get a quick nap then we can go together? I am afraid you will get lost in all the huge trees," she said joking Susan. "You were asleep most all of the way, you even missed town."

It took Susan several minutes to convince Stephanie that she could handle it, and that, she would not get lost.

"Well as long as you give me some good directions," she added with a playful laugh.

"Well, if you go to the end of the drive, make a left and go about seven miles there is a small town we passed through on the way here. I am sure you will be able to find some provisions there for us. I think maybe I should write it down for you just in case you forget it," Stephanie added.

"Stop it, I don't think I need them written down, I will remember them," Susan said, "go rest. I will find it and heck, with the On-Star we have in the car I cannot get lost anyway, remember? So stop worrying and get some rest. We are going to have a talk fest tonight over hot dogs and lots of marshmallows," she added with a smile, "that is if I can get out of here to go get them before dark, now go rest my dear," she said with a lingering kiss on Steph's soft full lips.

She had very little trouble finding the town other than one small wrong turn out of the drive and twenty-two miles later into the vast wilderness.

Seeing the river coming up before her with nothing but forest beyond that she decided On-Star was the way to go. She could not for the life of her remember what Stephanie had said, but she knew she should have been to the town by now.

As soon as the lady told her she had made a wrong turn about twenty-two miles back, she then remembered what Stephanie had said about turning left. She kicked herself all the way to town.

When she had gotten to the end of the long winding drive she had forgotten which way to go. All she saw both ways was nothing but forest. Seeing a clearing some miles up if she turned right she went with it since all she saw left was more trees.

Knowing Stephanie would be tickled and full of "I told you so's" if she found out, Susan was determined not to let her find out. When she was talking to the nice guy that answered her On-Star call after getting turned around and on the right track she casually asked him if they keep logs on all calls they received. She then had to tell him what happened, as he was curious as to why she asked that sort of question. As they laughed about it he assured her that he would hit the delete button right now so there would be no record of her call at all. It was a rental car, and if he didn't delete it off the computer screen when they turned the car back in it would show up when they printed their receipt out. He said he didn't want her to have to live it down. Thanking him, she bid him a great day and just smiled to herself the rest of the drive.

She found the little town charming to say the least. It was very quaint. And she had no trouble finding the store as everything was lined up on either side of the one-road town.

As she was shopping for the food for them, she soon realized that this was something she wanted to do for them often, even if it meant moving to where ever Stephanie wanted to move to.

She now knew beyond a shadow of a doubt that's what she wanted to do, she knew she loved this woman and would make it work out. She could not figure out why she had been fighting it so much.

The lady at the register was very nice and Susan found it refreshing. At home they were nice most of the time, but as it was a tourist town they tended to get cranky after one of the huge cruise ships would dock and the town was invaded. She could not really blame them; some of the people were great that came to the Keys, but others were nothing but rude.

As the older lady rang her up, Susan's mind wandered to when she had taking the Olivia lesbian only cruise with a friend a couple of years ago. She remembered how nice everyone was on that ship, but when they had docked in one of the other countries another ship was also in port when they got there, and those people were very rude to the people of the island. They didn't want anything to do with them and most of them did end up getting rude services and...

"Miss... Miss, I don't mean to bother you," Susan heard a voice say as the nice old lady was smiling at her, "but your total is $76.45."

"I am so sorry," Susan said, paying the woman. "We just drove here from Key West and I am tired. I guess my mind was just wondering off in la la land..."

The woman just smiled at her as Susan hurried out the door feeling very foolish. "This is another one of the new memories I will have to forget about, so I don't need to tell Stephanie," Susan thought to herself.

# CHAPTER 39

Stephanie was still asleep when Susan finally returned, and she was glad. This way she would not know it took her so long. She was as quiet as she could be when she put the supplies away. She had also gotten some charcoal for the grill not knowing if there was any there or not.

She was sitting on the patio outback letting the grill warm up; she closed her eyes and was listening to the Whippoorwills singing their night song when Steph walked out the side door.

"Hi sleepy-head," Susan said as Stephanie walked up beside her.

"You should have woke me up when you got home; I have slept most of the day away."

"Do you still have your headache? I remembered to grab some Aleve while I was in town, just in case it didn't go away with a nap."

"Nope it is all gone, but thank you honey that was so sweet of you," Stephanie offered. "All I needed was to rest. So did you have any trouble finding the town?"

"Who me?" Susan offered with an innocent smile creeping across her face. "It was a piece of cake," she finally said.

It didn't take long for the grill to heat up enough to cook their hot dogs, but it took a bit of time to actually get them on the grill because Stephanie challenged Susan to a sword match using hot dogs as their weapon of choice. Five wasted hot dogs later; Susan won. She then claimed her reward from the loser, which was a kiss on the cheek as they both giggled.

"I'm glad there is a little chill in the air; I think it helps keep the mosquitoes away," Susan said after they had finished eating. She took the last hot dog off the grill and broke it into little pieces for the squirrels to eat tomorrow.

"I'll go get the marshmallows," Stephanie said running into the cabin.

Susan made a huge mess all over Stephanie's face trying to feed the soft, melting, whitish brown, gooey marshmallows to her. She giggled as she pulled a roasted one apart and ended up missing her mouth and getting it on her nose. As Susan was leaning over and licking it off her nose, she saw Stephanie out of the corner of her eyes sneak the last one out of the bag.

"Hey, I saw that, no fair, you get more marshmallows than me and I am the one that went to buy them," Susan pretended to pout about it "It's a good thing I am too stuffed from so many hot dogs. I also wanted to say thank you for bringing me here, we did need this away time in a neutral place," Susan said as she cozied herself into Steph arms.

"I agree," Stephanie whispered as she started kissing Susan's neck and ear. "This is for kissing my nose," she said as she licked her neck "Oh, you taste like hot dogs and mustard," she added with a laugh, as she licked a small bit of mustard off her cheek, ".my favorite."

Giggling, Susan pulled back, "Ok, ok hold on there Ms. love machine, we are going to start talking tonight remember?"

"Ok," Stephanie pretended to be hurt, "let's talk, because then after we are done..." she didn't finish, she wanted Susan's mind to run wild. She added with an evil grin. "Who wants to go first?"

"Well why don't you, since I bet you have more energy as you had a lot more marshmallows than me," Susan said giggling.

"Oh you just think your too cute don't you?" she said pinching Susan's arm. "And it's a good thing that you are also or else. Well I have done a lot of thinking the whole drive up as a matter of fact, and I know I do love you and that no matter what I want to make it work. I would really love to open a ranch up on the mountain of some sort, together, with you, but not without you. I want you to be happy also. So what I was thinking that we could do would be to spend as many months as needed to get it up and running.  I think it will be a self-sustaining place for the most part, so I was thinking we could divide our time up between the two places. In the cold winter months that you don't care for we can live in Florida or anywhere else you want to live, and then in the summer we can be at the ranch.   Honey don't you think we could make that work, I just know we could if we tried."

Seeing tears in Susan's eyes, Stephanie grew worried. "Did I say anything wrong?" Stephanie wanted to know.

"No, not at all baby, these are my happy tears," Susan added. "I have been such a fool for so long and heck a little snow won't keep me from you. I was also thinking about the same things while I was in town getting the food, wherever you are, is where my heart will be so. We can do it together. I'll sell the boat and pack up and…"

"Now wait a minute," Stephanie cut in, "if you are going to learn to like snow, the least I can do is learn to like the ocean, sand, and the house boat. If nothing else I will buy stock in the Dramamine Company to help me get through," she added with a smile. "I want to take the next week and build on what we have started already, then we can go get the ball rolling on the rest. What do you say?"

"I would say that sounds so wonderful, it's a start to our perfect plan," Susan said. "This is going to be our week."

"Not too perfect I hope," Stephanie added, "we need to leave some room for faults. I know I have one or two faults myself."

"Don't we all have some of those?" Susan said, "Don't we all?"

"Hey you know what would be good right now?" Stephanie said as she stood up and stretched. "I am thinking a nice night swim," and as she took off running she yelled, "I'm going to beat you this time, and I want a back rub when I do!"

As Susan chased after her she saw that Stephanie was already in the water splashing around. When she got to the lakes edge she started pulling off her clothing, she went to the edge to test the water with her toe.

"Hey, how did you get undressed so fast?" Susan wanted to know. Stephanie just laughed and tried to splash her.

"You are nuts," Susan said as she stuck her toes into the water. "This water is freezing," pulling her toes back out quickly. "If you want a back rub that bad, you got it. I give in, I'm not getting into that ice water," she added with a laugh.

"It's ok if you're a big sissy baby Susan, but I do plan on collecting on my back rub tonight." Stephanie added with fits of laughter, "I won't forget," she yelled as Susan was grabbing her clothing she had discarded along the trail.

"Oh I'll give you one all right, and don't think I will be stopping with just the back," Susan laughed.

"Good," Stephanie said with a wink, "I was hoping for a lot more."

The days and nights melted together as they made love and talked and grew closer. They both love the nature hikes and exploring. No matter how hard Steph tried the whole time they were there she could not get Susan to go for a cold night swim though.

"I hate that this time of ours has went by so dang fast, but this past week has been wonderful," Susan cooed. "I have had the most wonderful and relaxing time here. Hey, I have an idea," she added.

"What would that be dear?"

"Well, I thought maybe on our way to Colorado we could make a little detour and hit the state of Vermont and..."

"Vermont? Why there?" Stephanie asked.

"Well I was thinking that we might find a quaint little chapel, and maybe say an I do or two and start the ranch as a married couple even if it will only be legal in Vermont, we will know we are married. So what do you say Steph?"

"Well your mind has been working over time I see," Stephanie said after she thought about it a few minutes. "I like the idea and all honey, but I have a few things when we get back to Colorado that needs to be taken care of first. If it isn't I don't think it will be fair to you, and I think also we should drive back to the Keys and get you some things packed and lock the houseboat up. I sort of thought if we got married at the ranch even if it wasn't legal it would be to us, and I sort of think that would be even more special. I think you need to let your work know also that you won't be there, right?"

"Well I forgot to tell you that when you threw me out, so you could make plans, I had a talk with Ms. Ellen. I let her know I was not sure what was going to happen for this

285

coming school year and not to plan on me being there. As always you're correct honey, we need to get the other things squared away in Florida first. To tell you the truth I do like the marriage on the mountain idea, it is a good thing one of us has a good head on their shoulders," Susan added. "Marriage is something that we both want isn't it?" Susan said, a little unsure of Steph's answer.

"More than anything baby, more than anything," Stephanie said. "I just want us to have everything going, and I want us both to be settled in."

They both stood looking back at the cabin and woods after all their bags were in the car, neither wanted to leave but both wanted to go so they could get the plans they had made rolling.

Steph's head was working overtime as she had a plan in the works that she didn't tell Susan about; it was going to be a surprise for her birthday in November. Proud of herself for coming up with it, she wrapped her arms around Susan's shoulders and led her to the car.

"Lets go honey, we've got our life ahead of us," with that they both had to laugh.

The drive back to the Keys was a nice, pleasant one, except when they ran into some rain outside of Melbourne. It had been a mad dash to pull over and get the top put up on the car before they got totally soaked, this time Susan stayed awake to keep Stephanie Company.

As they got back to the Keys the weather was a little nasty, it had not started to rain yet but Susan knew it would not be long before it blew in as the hurricane had moved closer to Florida. She was hoping to get everything shut up before it hit. Susan assured Stephanie that there was nothing to worry about. They had weather like this each year during this season, but Stephanie didn't feel reassured at all and she was relieved that she had talked Susan into moving with her where they were safe away from the ocean.

As Susan came out with the last bag she was taking with her she looked at Stephanie standing at the end of the pier. The wind was blowing her hair, and Susan got lost in daydreaming about Stephanie for a minute.

"All done," Susan called out to her. "Are you ready for me to call a taxi?"

"I think so," Stephanie said a little perplexed, then she added "are you sure your place will be ok? The water seems to just toss the boats back and forth."

Smiling at her, Susan assured her it would be fine.

"The packing up and closing up process took a lot less time than I figured it would," Stephanie said. "Thank goodness you're a light packer," she said as she came over to help carry the last of Susan's bags to the taxi. "At least with not so many bags, but the ones you do have sure are heavy."

"Hey just because you can live in jeans and a flannel shirt every day of your life doesn't mean you need to chain me to that way of dressing," Susan jabbed at Stephanie, "I had to pack for winter weather also, remember?"

"Yes, but how much does some sweaters weigh and this old winter jacket?" she said as she was laying it in the trunk. She pretended the bags were too heavy, and she couldn't lift them up into the truck, and that she was now too tired to carry another bag.

"If I didn't love you so much," Susan started to say giggling, but stopped as she saw the rolling of the cabbies eyes, "I think he wants to get going," Susan whispered to Stephanie.

Giggling, both women got the entire stack of bags in the trunk, and Stephanie watched as Susan hugged everyone that had showed up to see them off. As she climbed into the car she blew them all kisses, promising to call after they got there and got settled in, and off they went to the airport.

They were lucky enough this time to get seats together, as the plane was more than half empty. When they got to their seats Susan had to switch because they had given Stephanie the window seat on accident and she was too afraid. Susan had tried to get her to look out the window during the flight to Florida, but that was a lost cause.

"I guess no one wants to be going towards the cold weather," Susan said. "Well at least that is what that really nice guy at the airport in Colorado that wouldn't let us sit together said when we took the flight here to Florida," Susan said with a giggle.

"Oh you're funny, speaking of nice guys didn't you forget to tell me something? I almost forgot to mention something about it," Stephanie began, "for some reason I think you forgot to tell me something now didn't you?"

A worried look came over Susan as she tried to figure out what she had left out or forgotten to tell her; then she felt a little relieved when Stephanie started laughing.

"What's so funny?" Susan wanted to know.

"Well it seems that when I turned the rental car in I had an extra charge on the bill that someone forgot to tell me about," she could see Susan was lost so she went on. "Well, it seems that each time you call On-Star there is a charge, and I think someone forgot to mention they had gotten lost their first day there and tried to get some nice guy there to cover for them," she added, laughing from the look on Susan's face.

"I cannot believe you found out and that guy was so nice, he said he was going to delete it, I cannot believe he did that, it serves me right I guess." Susan said in a fit of giggles. "You will never let me live it down now will you? See if I ever call On-Star again. Next time I will drive to Tim buck two first and just stay lost before I will ever call them."

Stephanie was laughing so hard tears were running down her face as the passengers in other seats looked back at them.

"I was so hoping they were right and you did use it and it wasn't just a mistake on their part. You know I have to give you a little grief over it," she added a smile to that last statement.

The flight was a long one. Most of the passengers were asleep when Stephanie leaned over to Susan and whispered in her ear.

"You want to join the club?" she asked as quiet as she could.

"What are you talking about?" Susan wanted to know.

Stephanie was trying not to giggle as she grabbed the blanket from overhead and spread it across them both. She leaned over and kissed Susan and said, "The mile high club, silly."

Susan got a knowing look in her eyes as she felt Steph's hand slip under the covers and up her leg. Susan looked around quickly to see if anyone could see them. When she was sure they were all asleep she leaned over and started kissing her, whispering she said, "You don't even like to fly. How do you know about this club?" she added with a giggle.

"I may not like to fly but I like to read and I have heard a story or too, and, I want to join up, do my part to make the friendly skies friendlier," she added with a snicker.

Both women had a problem with being loud during sex so it was all they could do to keep it down. They both had their hands down the others pants stroking each other under the cover trying not to make too much noise. Susan was the first to reach the point of no return. As her body grew stiff she had to muffle herself in Steph's shoulder to keep from crying out. Seeing Susan cum sent Steph over the edge.

Susan leaned over and kissed Stephanie's nose. "I love you baby," she whispered as she laid her head on her shoulder and decided to try and get some rest before they landed.

Stephanie woke up when the pilot came over the loud speaker and announced they would be landing in Colorado Springs in five minutes. The landing was a smooth one and for that Susan was grateful; she was worried that if it were too rough she would not be able to get Stephanie back on a plane.

As they were departing the plane they happened to be the last passengers off as they were seated all the way in the back. When they got to the front where the flight attendants stood to greet and say good-bye to everyone, one of the attendants looked them in the eye and said, "Congratulations."

Susan looked at Stephanie to see if she knew what the lady was talking about. Seeing she was just as lost she asked, "Congratulations? Congratulations for what?"

"For joining the mile high club, of course," the flight attendant said with a wink to them both.

Both ladies could not stop from turning red and giggling all the way up the ramp as they hurried to get as far away from the attendants as they could.

It took Susan a while to locate all the bags as Stephanie went to look for a cart to haul the bags on; they were both worried trying to remember where they had parked the jeep.

Thirty minutes later they had decided to split up to cover more ground in their search for the Jeep. It didn't take long before Susan yelled out that she had found it.

"I'm ready," Susan cut into Steph's thoughts.

"Ready?" Stephanie asked, "Ready for what babe?"

"Well, we are in the Springs and I am ready to go pick the rest of my things up and say my good-byes, this way we can start fresh with nothing hanging over us at all."

"Well then what are we waiting for?" Stephanie said with a faked lightness to her voice. She was trying not to worry about what might happen as soon as Susan saw Tiffany again.

"Come on," Susan said taking her hand, "it will be ok," she assured her. "Trust me." She could see the worry in Stephanie's eyes and she wanted to reassure her that she had nothing to worry about at all.

"Famous last words," Stephanie thought but she didn't say anything as they made their way to Tiffany's house.

They both rode in silence most of the way, lost in their own thoughts about the pending meeting with Tiffany.

"Guess it wasn't such a good idea," Susan said, seeing that no one was home, "just my luck that she wouldn't be home, some other time I guess."

"Wait a second honey, why don't you leave her a note with our phone number. So she can let us know when would be a good time for her for us to come by to get your things."

"You're a sweetheart," Susan said, "That's a good idea. That way we won't bother her or come when she isn't home again next time," she added.

They had a hard time finding something to write the note on. Stephanie found an old empty envelope so Susan jotted out the note on the back of it.

# CHAPTER 40

Susan couldn't help but noticed all the newspapers stacking up on the front porch as she stuck the note in the door. She tried to look through the window but she could not see anything.

"That's funny," Susan, remarked more to herself than to Steph as she got back in the Jeep.

"What is it honey, is there something wrong?" Stephanie asked a bit worried at Susan's reaction.

"Oh sorry," Susan said, "I guess I was talking out loud again, I tend to do that at times. It's just that there's several days worth of newspapers piled up on the porch and the mailbox is running over. It looks as if no one has been here in days. What I can't figure out is why Mable isn't coming over to take care of these things if Tiffany went away or something. I do hope she is ok. I don't think her mother has stayed away because of the weather, because the snow is almost gone and the roads are all clear. I don't think it has snowed here much since we left, so I know she could make it over here."

"Do you know where her mother lives?" Stephanie asked, "We could go over there and have a talk with her, I am sure she can reassure you that all is ok."

"I have no idea where she lives and I think we have done all we can do for now. I'm sure she will call when she gets home and has some free time," Susan added, "I think we should get on the road now though so we can get home before it gets dark."

"I like that very much," Stephanie said as she gave Susan's hand a little squeeze.

Looking at Stephanie she asked, "What do you like honey?"

"I like hearing you say home. It is our home now you know, I hope you feel that way also."

"What are you doing?" Susan asked as Stephanie pulled the Jeep over, they had just pulled out of Tiffany's drive.

"I was thinking that maybe you should drive the rest of the way to "our" house this time," Stephanie said.

"I don't like to drive most of the time, but I think that this time it would be a great idea," Susan said.

They drove in silence for a while, until Stephanie said "I think I will call Robert first thing when we get home and get an appointment set up for us as soon as he can fit us in, I don't think there is any reason to wait, do you? I want us to decide all things together now."

"I think that you're right. I don't think we need to wait at all, the sooner we start with the plans the sooner we finish. Now sit back and enjoy the ride my dear."

It didn't take Stephanie long to fall asleep, as Susan looked over at her sleeping next to her on the front seat she felt at ease, even Stephanie's little snores didn't bother Susan. She knew she had no doubts about them at all.

As Susan was driving up the mountain roads she realized that this was the first time since she had came back to this state that she didn't feel angry inside and she felt this was the first step to getting over her past hurts.

"Hey baby, wake up we're here," Susan announced touching Steph's face, brushing the hair back from her forehead awaking her.

"I fell asleep?" Stephanie asked. "It sure makes the trip seem a lot shorter doesn't it? I am so sorry you had to make the last leg of it alone."

"Why yes you did fall asleep, some time back in fact. And don't be sorry at all, I liked it. Anyway, you always get the fun of seeing me sleep, with my mouth open I am sure," she added, "and I never get to watch you, so it was all my pleasure."

"I liked it every time you would fall asleep when I was driving," she said smiling at Susan.

It didn't take them long to get all the suitcases and bags in. The wind was picking up and it felt as if a storm was trying to blow in. "Oh great, I see how it is," Susan said, "it has been pretty weather here for two weeks while we were gone and the moment I get back to town there is a storm brewing. Shoot, I don't remember which suitcase I packed my love for the snow in," she added with a giggle. Stephanie just smiled at her.

"I am going to give Robert a call while you get your things put away," Stephanie said, showing Susan which was her closet and which dressers she would be using.

"All done," Stephanie said hanging up the telephone and coming into the room, "we have an appointment at 10:00 in the morning. So don't make any other plans," she joked.

"I'm surprised that we got an appointment that quick, and just for you I do think I can keep tomorrow free. Now let's get ready for bed woman, we have a long day ahead of us. Many new things begin tomorrow," Susan said, taking Stephanie by the hand. "How about a nice long hot bubble bath together?" she added with a wink.

As they cuddled that night Susan sighed loudly.

"Is there anything wrong?" Stephanie wanted to know.

"No sweetness that was only a sigh of relief, nothing bad at all. I am just very satiated, and I am for once in a long time very happy and the good part is that it is here with you."

"I like that word," Stephanie said, "I think it describes how we both feel in a positive way. Now go to sleep woman unless you want me to keep you up half the night again that is."

Early the next morning as Stephanie rolled over she found the bed empty and cold next to her; she got worried about Susan and went to the living room looking for her.

Stephanie stood in the doorway and watched her for a minute. Susan was sitting on the end of the couch with her legs curled under her, lost deep in thought.

"I see you are up early this morning. Did you have another of your bad dreams? I am here if you want to talk about it you know?"

"Yes, I know you are here for me baby, it is just that I have so much on my mind it was hard to sleep, and then I did have a little bit of a bad dream," Susan offered, "when I woke up you just looked so peaceful and I wanted to let you sleep in a bit. It is still really early, so I got up, afraid I would wake you if I stayed in bed."

"It is a big day honey," Stephanie offered, "I am sure that with everything else that was weighing heavy on your mind it was hard for you to sleep. Let me get a good fire going, and maybe, if you want to talk and tell me about your dream you can, I would like that. Now you will need to kiss me, with my morning breath and all," she added with a giggle. "I am here for you honey on everything, as I told you."

"Your morning breath is a little bad this morning maybe it isn't such a good trade off. Let me think here, warm fire or yucky kisses," she teased. "I will share my dreams with you later. I like to think about it and process it first if that is ok, and I love it when you do that."

"What's that honey?" Stephanie wanted to know.

"I love your giggle, no matter what mood I am in when I hear your giggle I feel a smile coming on. You just have a way with my mood and heart, you lighten them both up."

"Well good," Stephanie said. "Cause I tend to giggle a whole lot now days it seems, all due to you of course," she added with a wink.

Stephanie busied herself making a roaring fire, as she stood up she could see that Susan was deep in thought again.

"I have a feeling your mind is not on our meeting today," Stephanie said interrupting Susan's thoughts.

"I'm sorry honey. I don't mean to space out on you, I guess I am just a little worried about Tiffany and her mother. It is hard for me to just cut feelings off, and well, I am sorry. I don't mean to be thinking about all this, something just didn't seem right when we were there is all."

"No," Stephanie cut in, "nothing to be sorry about at all, you're a tenderhearted person and that is one reason I love you as much as I do. I am sure all is fine. I think Tiffany just took her mother on a vacation, she has had a rough few weeks herself. You know she needed to get away, and well, if it was spur of the moment it was probably just poor planning on their parts with asking someone to take care of picking up the newspaper and mail and such, ok?"

Susan was relieved that Stephanie wasn't mad at her, and she shook her head that she agreed with her.

"Ok then, stop worrying so much. I am sure things are fine."

"I know. You're right I'm sure," Susan said. "If it was anything I would have had a message when we got back to Florida, so I know all is ok, and now I am truly going to put it out of my mind and put my mind here where it goes. Thank you for not being mad and also for being so understanding about it all. Tiffany and her mother did both said they needed to get away on a long vacation during brunch that day."

"Well see then," Stephanie, said satisfied with herself.

The morning turned out to be beautiful. The storm blew over without so much as a hint of snow or rain, and they both decided to get an early start as they were up already. After they showered, they headed out the door to town.

"You know what this town reminds me of? This is just like all the little towns you see on TV," Susan said, "I feel like I am on the show Mayberry as I walk down the street with everyone waving at us like they know us. I really like that, people are friendly in Key West, don't get me wrong, but here it is so different, even homely in a good way though."

"That's one thing I love about it here, it has always felt like home no matter where I was in my life. I don't think anyone here has ever met a stranger here. Just wait, you'll see honey, the more you are here around all of this the more you will feel just like you have a bunch of grandparents and new best friends. Everyone is so excepting of everyone else also, I don't think there is a person in this town that doesn't know about my sexuality, and I have never had any trouble at all. I think that is what makes me so open, I have never had to hide it here."

"I can so tell what you mean. Thank you," Susan whispered. "Thank you for bringing me here and sharing all this with me."

Stephanie just pulled her close and kissed her. She was glad she had her here to share it with. She was very proud of Susan and wanted to show her off.

As they got to a little drug store that had a bench out front Susan was feeling a little lightheaded, "hey dear lets rest here for a few minutes."

Growing concerned Stephanie asked, "Are you feeling ok? You do look a little pale right now. Here lets rest here first and then we will go."

After a few minutes of resting Susan was feeling better

"Come on dear," she said. "I feel much better. I think I should not have skipped breakfast. I have sort of gotten use to you cooking for me in the mornings," she added with a smile. "Hint, hint."

# CHAPTER 41

Stephanie was still a little worried about Susan as she showed her around town. She pointed out all the little antique shops and all the homemade stuff stores. Susan could tell that she was proud of this town. They ended up getting to Robert's office a little early and he wasn't in so they decided to sit out front and wait for him to get in.

"The air is a bit brisk this morning but it is so lovely out here today," Susan said as she grabbed Steph's hand.

"Hello ladies," Robert said, "come in, come in. Grab a seat, sorry I am a bit late, I stopped by to grab us some doughnuts and bagels. You know Thelma, she could talk your ear off if you let her," he said smiling at Susan, "just wait until you meet her," he said. "Ok lets get started. First off, I took the liberty to have some specs drawn up after we talked last night. I also have a contractor and an accountant coming to this meeting in a few minutes, just going off what you told me on the phone last night that you two would like to do. I figured we could go over it all again this morning and before they get here though I thought we could get these contracts all signed and ready to go. Here you are Susan," he said as he handed her a stack of paper and an ink pen.

"Wow this is a lot of paper work. What is all this?" Susan asked looking at all the forms in front of her, Susan saw Robert look at Stephanie as if to say, "tell her."

"Honey," Stephanie started, "this is my surprise to you. I thought before we do anything we get all this legal, so I asked Robert to get all the deeds and all the financial information ready for you to sign. I want this to be ours, so therefore I am giving you half of everything."

"Oh no, I cannot do that Stephanie, Miss Rose, left it to you. I would not feel right about it. I thought I was just going to share in the Bed and Breakfast plans with you. Getting it built and up and running. I don't know about all this other stuff."

"Honey, she left it all for my future and you are my future. I assure you this is what she would have wanted. She has always hoped I would find someone like you that I wanted to spend my life with, trust me this is what she would want; I know she is smiling down at us right now. Now that said come on woman," she joked, "sign."

As Susan was looking over the contracts, Stephanie could tell she was still very hesitant, "When we marry I would expect to have half of everything you have as that is the law, and I would expect you to have half of everything of mine also."

"Well half of mine is nothing more than a houseboat, a small savings account and a small stack of credit card bills.

Nothing like all this, what all are we talking here Robert?" Susan asked looking up at him.

"Well, as you can see from the files in front of you," Robert began coming over to stand by her pointing out certain figures on different pages, "the size of the estate is substantial. With all the acreage of land, as well as the stocks and bonds and the bank accounts, we are talking in the millions; these contracts will give you both a fifty-fifty share."

"OH MY GOD!" Susan said, "No way can I do this that is just way too much to digest all at once. I just do not feel comfortable with all this; it is just so fast Stephanie. Can we please talk about this more before we decide?"

"Honey, we did talk about it, and we want to be together so this is just the next step."

"I know," Susan said, "but you did not tell me what all was included. I thought some land was the extent of it. This is just way too much."

"I don't mean to interrupt you both but I think I have a solution to all this," Robert cut in, "I will write it into the contract that you will have up to ninety days in which to change your mind and have your name taken off all the contracts, holding you not responsible for anything if you so choose to do that. This way you have plenty of time to think about it and talk more about it. I agree with you that it is a lot to digest all at once for anyone. So what do you think?"

Susan was still a little perplexed about the whole thing but shook her head yes, to give him the go ahead. "I think I can deal ok with that plan," she said smiling at Susan.

About the time Susan got all the papers signed, Robert's secretary buzzed him to let him know the rest of the group was there and ready to join the meeting.

"I think we're all ready for them now," Robert said into the intercom, "send them in and please bring us some coffee also.

After all the introductions were made and a few jokes exchanged between everyone, they decided to get down to business as no one wanted to be there all day.

Emerging outside Robert's office over three hours later both women felt drained and exhausted.

"I am starving," Susan said, "how about we go get some lunch before heading home?"

"I know just the place, I am a little hungry myself," Steph said with a twinkle in her eye.

"Oh no you don't," Susan said, "I'll pick the restaurant, you will have me singing for my lunch this time, and I am too tired for karaoke today," she added with a smile. "I think I have cramps in my hand from signing my name to too many papers today."

"Hand cramps, that's a likely story," Stephanie said. "You're just trying to get out of singing again," she added with a laugh.

As they were walking Susan saw a quaint little restaurant tucked in the back of a little store that she decided they were going to eat at.

"I think we should go over all this again," Susan said over lunch, "I am still a little taken a back with it all. It is all moving so fast, so let me get this straight. Come Monday all the contractors, developers and landscapers as well as most of the rest of the town is going to meet us first thing out at the site?"

"Yep that's right," Stephanie said with a proud smile. "Why wait? When we can get it going now and by the fall I hope we can have it at least ready to get the caretaker in it, if you don't want to live there. I think it will be a nice mountain retreat, a get away if you will, and I know it will bring a lot of much needed business to this little town."

"A B&B of sorts, for lesbians? How quaint."

"Yes for lesbians," Stephanie said smiling, "as well as others, all will be welcome. We will be everyone friendly."

"I like that better than to just cater to one type of people, do you think we will be able to get enough business up here to keep it running? It is sort of out of the way."

"Heck yes, there will be more business than we will know what to do with most of the time. We are in a remote location and people love that. In the winter we can have anything from skiing to other winter things for them to do, and the summer will be as much fun also, with horseback riding on some of the trails to hiking in the mountains. I will let you take care of the planning of things for people to do, and I took all sorts of marketing and business classes in college. I will start first thing next week getting the word out. The contractors said this morning that they think a solid three months of good weather and non-stop working and we should be ready to start decorating."

"I must admit that I am kind of excited about all this, it all seems so fast but exciting. I really enjoy having something to do." Susan said with a sparkle to her eyes that Stephanie had not seen before.

After a full day of talking and planning with Robert and more talking and planning over lunch and a visit later to the bank, they decided to stop in the bakery for some crescent rolls for the next morning.

"Come on, I want to introduce you to Thelma; Robert was right she will talk your ear off though. You will love her she is a sweet old woman; she makes the most wonderful baked goods around. I think I will talk to her about being our baker for the B&B so we can offer fresh goodies to our boarders."

While Susan was standing there talking to Thelma, making plans for after they were up and running, Susan began feeling light headed again. She started to sway back and forth as a wave of nausea and hot flashes came over her. She had to grab onto the edge of the counter to keep from falling over, this spell was worse then any of the others had been and she was worried.

"Stephanie, I'm sorry to interrupt you but I think we should head for home. I am so tired; I am just feeling drained and even a bit light-headed. I don't know why, I didn't even do anything strenuous. Maybe it is all this newness or stress, who knows, but I want to go home if you don't mind. It is getting late anyway and I think I should turn in early." She didn't want to worry Steph.

"Ok sweetness, let's head back before it gets any later, it has been a long day. Bye dear," she said to Thelma. "We'll talk more later."

"It was lovely to meet you," Thelma said hugging Susan, "I wouldn't worry about being light-headed too much dear. It is probably just this high elevation as to why you are feeling so tired and drained. It takes some getting use to being up here, even my ears pop still at times and I have lived up here for sixty-four years," she added with a smile. "Your blood will thin out soon and you'll feel like your old self or better in no time flat."

"Probably," Susan agreed, "I had not even thought of that. It was so nice to meet you also. Everything in here smells so great. If I had not just had a big lunch I would be sampling everything. I promise to eat plenty of all this you put in the bag in the morning."

After they got home, Stephanie said, "I will run you a bath, then I'll make us some tea to drink while you're in the tub. I think some lemon tea will hit the spot nicely, don't you?" she could tell that Susan wasn't feeling very well at all now.

"Thank you, I think you might be right," Susan added with the best smile she could manage.

As Stephanie brought the tea in she could see Susan had fallen asleep in the tub, "Come on honey," she said helping her out of the tub and into bed, "I am going to get in some wood and then I'll be right back in, try to get some rest."

Susan was already sound asleep when Stephanie was finished with the wood and her bath; she was feeling pretty tired herself and went right off to sleep.

Some time in the wee morning hours, Susan bolted straight up in the bed, sweating and shaking all over, waking Stephanie.

"What is it Susan? Susan?" Getting no answer she touched Susan's shoulder to gently shake her awake, Susan jerked away and screamed.

# CHAPTER 42

"You're ok honey," Stephanie kept trying to assure her, "it was just a bad dream baby, only a dream. Are you ok?" Steph felt helpless as she watched Susan sat there slumped over crying, "Honey talk to me," Stephanie pleaded, "I don't know what to do."

After a few minutes Susan said, "It was horrible, just awful. I don't want to talk about it. Hold me," she sniffled. "Please just hold me," she begged Stephanie as she lay back down to cuddle into her arms.

Stephanie lay awake for a long time not knowing what else to do other than just to hold her. She felt helpless, she knew very little of Susan's past.

She could tell the dreams were becoming worse and a lot more frequent, "Maybe it is this state and all its ghost memories that haunts her," Steph thought as she finally drifted off to sleep.

The next morning Susan made no mention of the episode from last night, and Stephanie wondered if she even remembered it. Somehow she knew she did.

After a couple of days when Susan didn't feel much better she decided to make an appointment with the doctor in the Springs to have a check up. She didn't want Stephanie to worry so she didn't tell her about it.

She made an excuse of why she would be gone for the day and then took off. Steph was busy with the builders anyway and thought nothing of it.

As she sat in the doctor's office after her check up waiting for him to come in she got up the courage to ask him for a referral for a good therapist, as the dreams were getting worse. She was beginning to lose control of them and she didn't like being out of control.

As the doctor came back into his office she could tell something was wrong. She left his office forgetting to ask for a referral, she knew she had to get up the courage to tell Stephanie about what he said. "If I can," she thought.

Several days went by before any more bad dreams happened. When it did Stephanie decided to brooch the subject with Susan about it, as she was growing more concerned.

"You had sort of another bad night last night didn't you honey? I was hoping that maybe you and I could sit and talk about it."

"I am sorry. Did I keep you awake? I could sleep on the couch from now on if you would like," she offered.

"No way, don't be silly I just was wondering if you wanted to talked about it, if you thought it might help you. You know what they say that if you get it out it often times helps."

"No thank you," Susan said, "I don't think it would help and anyway I don't remember most of them the next day," seeing Steph's non-believing look Susan added, "its true honey. They're so real when they happen, but by the morning, they are completely gone. I know they are all about the past but that is it, I don't remember nothing else, except feeling scared. Maybe I am not suppose to remember them or something," she offered.

"I am not buying it for a minute," Stephanie said, "but I will hold my tongue on it and just know I am here if you need to or just want to talk about it ok?"

Susan shook her head. "Ok. I do have something else I need to talk to you about though. A few days ago when I told you I had errands to do, I sort of lied, I did have an errand but the errand was a doctor's appointment that I had made. Ever since we got back I have not felt well as you know with being light headed and even my weight loss, I have been feeling light headed off and on for months now, so I made an appointment in the Springs and went and had a check up."

"Honey, I was very concerned about you. I am glad you went, but why didn't you tell me? I would have gone with you," Stephanie said even more concerned now. "What did he say?"

"Calm down, he said I need surgery soon, the sooner the better. He said that I have a cyst on my ovaries," as she got tears in her eyes it was hard to go on.

Seeing the concerned look on Steph's face she finished, "he said I would be fine honey, but he said I would never be able to have kids. That is if I ever wanted them. The worst part is he said from what he knows that it is hereditary, and that, he is sure I got it from my mother or her side of the family anyway. Wouldn't you know it, the only thing I ever got from them was something like this."

Stephanie went over and took Susan in her arms, "We are in this together honey and if we ever want kids we will just adopt, ok? Lets not worry about that at all right now. Lets get you well. When is the surgery?"

"In two days," Susan said. "He said it would take a few days to recover. But that they use lasers now and it isn't as evasive as it use to be."

"Well good then, we will have you up and running the builders in no time," Stephanie said with only a hint of worry showing in her voice.

The doctor turned out to be really nice and good at his job to Steph's relief. Susan was only a little scared going into surgery, at least on the surface, as Stephanie squeezed her hand and let her know she would be right there when she got out.

When the surgery was over the doctor came out to talk with Steph. He assured her Susan was doing fine and that once the anesthesia started wearing off and Susan started coming around, she would be able to go back and see her. She could take her home tomorrow if there were no complications, and he expected none.

313

The nurse came and got Stephanie a little while later when Susan woke up. She was groggy but not in much pain yet.

"Hi baby. Great news, I get to take you home tomorrow and the doctor said you will be up and around in just a few days."

"Good," Susan tried to say, "they won't let me have water and I am so dry," she whispered. "Ask the nurse for some ice chips please."

The nurse tried to make Stephanie leave when visiting hours was over but she would not. She sat by Susan's bed all night, sleeping with her head on the edge of the bed when she got too tired and could not stay awake any longer.

"Hi baby," Susan said as Stephanie woke up. She had been watching her sleep for a long time. "You sure didn't look very comfortable sleeping like that."

"I'm ok. I just wanted to be here with you. Don't you worry about me, ok?"

As Susan was about to say something the doctor came in.

"Morning ladies, I hear tell from the nurses that you are doing great and are ready to go home," he said to Susan, "and I hear you gave them grief last night young lady," he said to Steph. "But I'll forgive it this time," he said with a smile.

After he finished checking everything, he smiled at Susan and said, "By signing the papers you're a free woman, but you better hurry and get out of here or else they may find something else wrong," he joked.

"You don't need to tell us twice," Stephanie said. "I will go pull the Jeep around while you get dressed," she said to Susan as she kissed her and shook the doctors hand thanking him.

After she was gone, the doctor sat down on the edge of the bed and took Susan's hand in his. "I know this is hard on you," he said, "even if you were never planning kids at all this is a tough thing to go through. Here is a number I want you to call if you ever feel like you need to talk about this or anything else, she is really a great therapist. She is also a lesbian, and she is a very nice lady so keep her in mind and don't lose her card. I'll see you back in three weeks unless you need anything before then."

"Thank you doctor, you have been great, and thank you for this," she said, looking at the card, "I just may use it if for nothing more than some past demons that keep wanting to haunt me," she added with a smile.

Susan was a little uncomfortable on the drive back but it wasn't bad. They stopped at the drug store to get the medications she needed and then they were on their way home.

"Thank you baby," Susan said, "for just being there for me and with me. It means more than you could ever know."

The next few days were quiet. When she knew she felt well enough to get around she didn't want to stay in bed any longer. Feeling much better, she was ready to take on the task of being boss to the builders, or so she pretended.

Much of the next couple of weeks after Susan was back to normal were spent on the site during the days and making love and just spending time together at night, growing closer to one another as the days went by.

Neither one thought much of anything else other than the progress that was going on at the building site. The worry over Tiffany was also long gone.

Even if they were neither one much help they felt like they were helping by being there, overseeing everything. More in the way than helping, some of the workers might say as neither one knew the first thing about building anything at all.

"Hey guys want some help I am pretty sure I remember how to swing a hammer?" Susan offered, "I did make a birdhouse in shop class a long time ago, I think it was in the seventh grade. I'm sure I remember some of it anyway," she said with a laugh.

"Sorry ma'am," one of the cute guys said with a laugh, "but I am pretty sure that would not qualify you for much in the way of building your home here, unless you want to make a bird house to put up in that big old nice tree in the front yard, but then again it has been a long time. I am not sure if you would even remember how even," he said laughing.

"Ma'am? I cannot believe you called me that, what am I, old?" She said to the cute young worker, "Hush now," Susan said getting that familiar blush to her cheeks again, "you might just be surprised at what I can do, and I plan on having many birdhouses around the place," she added with a smile. "But I am good with a hammer."

"Here, prove it to them honey," Stephanie said holding out a hammer to her as a challenge, "show these men and me what my baby can do, come on darling make then eat their words," she teased.

Susan looked around and saw all the workers looking at her now. "Oh maybe another time, you know how fragile egos can be. They're doing such a wonderful job themselves I don't want to show them up and have them hurt and pouting we would never get any work done that way," she offered softly laughing even redder now as they all had fits of giggles themselves.

They all had a good laugh on what Susan said over a glass of ice tea Stephanie had brought up to the site for all the workers.

# CHAPTER 43

"Good morning baby girl, look what I have for you," Mable said coming into the little room carrying a big box.

"Oh Mom what is it?" Tiffany said as best as she could. Talking was still very hard for her as was most everything else.

"I'm not telling, you will just need to open it yourself and see," her mom said with one of her huge plastered on smiles that she put on and wore each day as she came into Tiff's room.

"I am so thankful you came to stay with me," she said trying to make her fingers grab hold of the ribbons on the box. Tiffany said to her mom, "I don't know what I would have done these last couple of months without you here with me mom, I don't think I would have even made it."

"Hush now, don't you talk like that. You know I've got to be with you baby girl, and heck I have gotten to see all sorts of new things here in this country, now open your gift," she added when she heard the whimpering coming from inside the box.

"What have you gone and done?" Tiffany wanted to know. "Is this something we are going to get in trouble for?" she asked as she felt the box move.

As she struggled to open the box her mother's first instinct was to rush over to help her out, but she

318

remembered what the doctors had told her. She knew they were right, Tiffany had to learn to do things on her own in her own way now or else she would become even more depressed, and there would be no pulling her back.

"Oh Mom!" Tiffany squealed as she saw the teeny, tiny puppy lying in the bottom of the box on the little blanket, looking up at her with big eyes and just the teensy whimper coming out of it.

"I love him!" Tiffany cried. "He is so small, can I hold him?" Then she grew worried, "Will they allow me to have him here with me?"

"It's not a boy it's a little girl," Mable said, "and yes, of course you may keep her here with you. I checked before I even got her and they're rules are nothing like back home, they don't mind at all. In fact they thought it a good idea because..." Mable didn't go on, she couldn't make herself even think that way, and she sure wasn't going to tell Tiffany that the doctors said she would never walk again, or ever be able to do much for herself. They felt that a little dog would lift her spirits if nothing more.

Tiffany was crying and happy now, not even listening to her mother anymore, "She is so little and so adorable. What kind of puppy is she mom?"

She is a cream colored mini-Pomeranian," her mother offered. "She will always stay little like this, she may get a pound or so bigger but not much at all. Isn't she so cute? When I saw her I knew she was the one for you."

"Well good morning ladies, what do we have here?" Warden Jones wanted to know.

At least that is what Tiffany called her and felt like she was most of the time when she was mean and made her do all the physical therapy that she didn't want to do.

"Hello Nurse Jones," Mable said, "I have checked with the doctor as well as others here on staff, and they felt that it was ok for Tiffany to have a puppy here with her while she is here. I am sorry but when I checked you weren't at work. I hope it is ok?"

"Well of course it is ok," Jones said, "and a cute thing it is too I see. If you are going to leave it over night love, you will need to have something worked out with the orderly to walk it for you," she said to Tiffany, "I'll be back in a little bit honey for your bath, and I need to change the catheter, but you can play with the puppy for a little bit first."

"Yes, of course, I understand, and I am sure I can get one of them to help me out," Tiffany said, tickled that she was able to keep the puppy here with her, "hey little one what are we going to name you?"

"Hold on," her mother said, "you can't name her."

"Why not?" Tiff wanted to know.

"Well my grandmother used to always say that all things had a name, just wait for it. She was an old wise Indian woman so I tend to agree with her; you just need to wait and see what her name is. Call her Baby for a few days while you watch her, and trust me, you will see what her

320

real name is suppose to be then in her mannerisms and actions."

"I think you're nuts mom but lets give it a shot, holding the puppy so she could look into its eyes she said I like calling her baby anyway," Tiffany said with a smile. "I have always wanted a puppy like this one but never thought I had time for one. Now look at me, I have nothing but time for one," Tiffany said, sad with tears in her eyes now.

Seeing Tiffany sad this way was almost more than she could stand, she had not seen her like this since her father died a year ago, not even when she lost Susan was she this sad. This was different and Mable didn't know if she would even pull through for sure. She tried to not let Tiffany see when she would get too sad or worried herself; she knew she had to be strong for Tiffany. It was going to be a long hard road to get her back health wise to the point where she could even go home.

The doctors all said there was no hope that she would ever walk again. The second blow, which she received to the back of the head saw to that, and the last blow to the spine sealed the deal when they kicked her in the back. They didn't know when she would be well enough to fly; they felt it would not be for months, maybe even a year.

All the many specialists that came in and saw Tiffany all most daily told Mable that they were lucky that she survived the attack at all and not to try and hurry anything along, it would happen when it was suppose to.

What upset Mable the most now was the fact that Tiffany grew more and more depressed each day; they would not release her to go home or give her any idea as to when they would. She felt trapped and helpless.

Mable knew they were just afraid that such a long flight back to the states would do more damage and they said with her being in a coma right after the attack they didn't want to chance a relapse. Her mother felt she could get her better care back home with her own doctors; she knew these were great doctors, but nothing was like home to Mable.

It didn't help matters, at least where Mable's feelings were concerned, when a lawyer told her that they might be afraid she was going to sue them. It made them nervous when a foreigner is attacked on their own soil by one of their own thugs.

"Mom?" Tiffany interrupted Mable's thoughts.

"Yes honey," her mother answered.

"Mom can we please talk? I want you to know Cindi and I were doing nothing wrong. I am so sorry I fought the attackers back. I don't remember much but I remember kicking back, maybe if I didn't fight back then they would have left us alone. I feel so guilty over it, what if I am the one that caused all this?"

"There is nothing to feel guilty over honey, you did the right thing. You did not cause anything, if you had not fought them at all you might not even be here," her mother said trying to hold back her own tears seeing Tiffany crying.

"I want to know about Cindi and what happened that day? I think I am strong enough to find out what happened, and how she is. I know you don't think so but I have got to know. All I do is lay here and think and worry about it, and I have got to know. When she asked me to go with her to her hotel to pack that day I said no, then I changed my mind and went with her. I didn't want her to have to go alone. I keep thinking I am such a fool for going. When Cindi and I were talking about making a fresh start while in this country we didn't know how right we were. Please mom, talk to me about it. I need to know how she is, the not knowing is so much worse than the knowing would be."

"Honey," her mother began, "I want for you to be able to remember everything in time, and I want you to know all about Cindi and what has…"

"Hello ladies," Ms. Jones said as she came back into the room, "I don't mean to disturb you both, but it is time for Tiff's bath and therapy." Looking at Mable the nurse said, "Why don't you go get a cup of coffee honey, and show the puppy off to all the patients? I think it will lift some spirits around here, just until we're done."

"Stop it; don't talk as if I am not even here," Tiffany said in an angry, defiant tone her mother remembered well from Tiffany's childhood.

"I'm sorry," Nurse Jones said, "I didn't mean to exclude you honey."

Mable was very thankful for Ms. Jones disturbance; she didn't want to brooch the subject with Tiffany about Cindi not now, not ever. She was doing her best to put the subject off the best she could. She knew her daughter, and she knew she would not give up, not until she got the information she wanted.

The doctors thought it best for her not to be told anything about Cindi being in a coma, and that she wasn't expected to make it at all. She had little to no brain activity and the prognosis was grim at best. They felt she would have too much guilt over the whole situation and therefore hinder her own recovery. They also felt that her mind was hiding the details of what happened that day for a reason and they were afraid that if the memories were triggered too fast it could send her right back into shock.

What they didn't know or even seem to understand was that she has so much guilt over not knowing what was going on that she could not even sleep.

She didn't remember much of the attack, but she knew they were walking and holding hands when several boys jumped them or men she didn't know which and that they had baseball bats and steel pipes.

Knowing Cindi had a family, made her feel even worse if that was possible. She so wanted to talk to Cindi to see how she was, she had point blank asked her mother if Cindi was dead and her mother had told her no. She knew her mother would not lie to her about it so that made her feel a little better, but she would not tell her anything else. She wasn't sure if her mother was afraid to let her know that maybe Cindi was in better shape than her or was she in even worse shape. Tiffany didn't know if that was even possible without them being dead, she thought as she was looking down at her ugly twisted, mangled body. She also wanted to talk to Cindi's husband and let him know that Cindi had done nothing to cause this attack, that she had done nothing wrong.

She remembered something the bobby had said to someone while he was at the hospital trying to investigate. That was when she was in and out of her coma, she remembered him talking to someone but she didn't know whom it was.

She didn't know anything at that point, not where she was or what had happened. She tried to open her eyes and speak to them, to ask someone, anyone, why she couldn't move, but her eyes wouldn't open and nothing would come out when she tried to talk.

Tiffany heard him say, as if he was way off in the distance, that he had talked to the hotel clerk and he said that he had given a statement to the fact that they were holding hands and flaunting it in front of everyone, and he felt that it was a bashing against them because of their sexuality.

She didn't know why, but she was sure then that he was talking about Cindi and herself. She wanted to scream out that they had not done anything wrong and that Cindi wasn't even gay, that they were just two people becoming great friends having fun being on vacation, but she could not move or even make her eyes open.

She remembered hearing nothing more for what seemed like a blink of an eye only, and which she learned later that it had been over a month. When she finally woke up and was able to open her eyes the first face she saw was her mother's tear stained face looking down at her.

"Mom," Tiffany whispered, "I thought I had dreamed that you were here. I heard talking at one point when I was half awake and thought someone said your name, but I didn't believe it was you," she said with tears in her eyes. Then it hit her where she was and that it must be something really serious if her mother flew all the way to Australia to be here with her.

"No honey it wasn't a dream I am really here; the doctor said at some point you might have been able to hear us. What do you remember hearing?" her mother asked.

"I don't remember anything really, other than just words that don't make any sense," Tiffany answered. "Was I in a car crash? Why can't I remember anything?" Tiffany said as she struggled trying to remember back "I wish I could remember what happened."

"The doctors said it might take some time to have all the memory come back, if they ever do at all. Just don't try to rush it," her mother added.

As Tiffany struggled to sit up her mother gently held her shoulder to lay her back down saying, "Lay down honey, let me call the nurse."

"Mom, why can't I move?" Tiffany cried, "I can't feel my legs," and then she noticed she could not feel her right hand or even talk plain either, "Mom what happened to me?" Tiffany started crying hard now.

"Yes?" the intercom buzzed as her mother pushed the button.

"Come quick Ms Jones, please hurry she is awake, my daughter, finally woke up," Tiffany could hear the relief in her mother's voice as she spoke to the little box.

Tiffany was very depressed for a few days after that and would not talk to anyone, not even Mable. The doctors told her she would never walk again and that she would be paralyzed on her right side also. They felt that she would, after several more surgeries, get most of her speech back. They could all tell that she was falling into a deep depression, and they didn't know how to stop it.

This was when her mother talked to them about getting a puppy for Tiffany; she had read that it help patients with these prognoses. She was relieved when they were all for the idea and thought as soon as she started to respond to treatment a little bit, that she could bring one in for her.

Tiffany slowly started coming around. She started asking more and more questions, many they had to avoid answering for her own good, and even started to try with the physical therapist in doing her exercises. Her mother felt this was a good time so she set out one day to find the perfect puppy for Tiffany.

When Mable walked into the room after Tiffany had had the puppy for several days, Tiffany said, "I have decided a name for her. I have watched her and you're right, she has her own name. I am going to call her Teffa for short but her name is Queen Latiffah."

Her mother laughed. "Why on earth did you come up with that name?" she wanted to know.

"Well," Tiffany began, "when she wants to go out for a walk she does this little moonwalk dance where she scrapes her feet backwards walking back as if she is really moon walking and does these baby barks. I found out last night when you're singing she tries to sing right along with you, it is so cute. I had the night nurse rolling with it. I was listening to one of Queen Latiffah's songs and singing along myself when she just started baby barking right along with me."

Her mother was still laughing as she shook her head picking up the puppy that was now showing off for her doing it's moon walking. "Teffa, hum, well Grandma likes it," she said, "so if you had been a male you would now be named

Michael Jackson I guess," she said laughing as she put Teffa on the bed next to Tiffany.

Mable was proud of Tiffany over the next couple months and so were the doctors. She made a better recovery than they had thought she would. They even talked about releasing her on a part time basis if she continued to keep improving as quickly as she was. She would still need to be there each day all day, but they were thinking about letting her out at night to go with her mother; they felt it would help life her spirits even more.

After Mable heard the good news she rented a small place next to the hospital when they had told her it would be at least eight months before they would think of releasing Tiffany to fly home. The place was ideal to get Tiffany back and forth to when they let her out of the hospital; it even had a wheelchair ramp at the back door. She knew it would help raise Tiffany's spirits even more to get her out of the hospital even for just the nights.

The hospital administrator had also asked Mable if she would be interested in helping to start a program for the other patients. He felt that having Teffa had helped Tiffany try harder in her recovery. He had also been told that she was in a deep depression before the puppy came to stay with her and that she snapped out of it quickly as soon as the puppy was brought in. So they had decided to give it a go with other patients. She would be handling and dealing with bringing animals in to help speed up the recovery of as many as they could. They decided to have a large room converted into a place to house the animals, and she would be in charge of the volunteers that would help her care for the animals and also take them around to see the different patients.

She knew she would be here for at least six more months so she agreed to help after she returned from the states, she had to make a quick run home as she had left so fast that she had forgotten to have someone house sit at both places as well as have the other things taken care of. She did feel it like it was a good cause and would work as she saw what a difference it made in Tiffany's attitude toward getting better. She was also thankful for something to help take her mind off some of Tiffany's pain.

When she told Tiffany about it she was ecstatic. She knew her mother needed something and she too thought it a great idea.

She became sad when Mable told her about her pending trip back home, "Honey it will only be for no more than a few days," she assured her. "I need to get everything settled back home then I will be right back. Is there anyone you would like me to contact?"

After thinking a few minutes Tiffany said, "Yes, please tell Larry. And let work know, I am sure they are all frantic with worry."

"I will take care of it honey, what about Susan?"

Looking down at her body she said, "No mom, I don't want her to know, no one else."

"Ok sweet heart."

She didn't know if she agreed with Tiffany but she would do whatever made her happy. "Now back to this animal plan here," mother said trying to get Tiffany's mind off that subject.

"Well, I for one think it is a wonderful idea, and it gives me something else to work for," she told her mother.

"What's that?" her mother asked.

"Well, when I get well enough I want to help you as much as I can with the animals, be your assistant," Tiffany said as she rubbed Teffa as she lay sleeping next to her.

"I think that is a wonderful idea," the doctor said coming into the room. "You will make a wonderful volunteer helping with the animals." Neither one of them had seen him standing there watching them.

# CHAPTER 44

The next three months flew by for Susan and Stephanie. Each pretty day was filled with being on site doing what they could do to help or at least get in the way. It made both of them feel as if the place was even more theirs, and on the rainy days they spent their time inside figuring out paints, wallpapers, carpet and other such things together.

"I love old things," Susan said, "I think we should do antiques everywhere we can."

"Great idea," Stephanie agreed, "I think they give a place such a comfortable, warm feeling. Did I ever tell you that was Rose's one passion in life? She loved her antiques, there is a house full of them of hers, well, ours now," she added a bit somber remembering back. Stephanie was so glad she had Susan here, she didn't think should could have handled Rose's death without her.

They decided they would go through the old house to see what they wanted to use for the new place. Susan felt funny being in a dead woman's house but didn't want Stephanie to have to go alone. It turned out to be a bigger project than either had anticipated it to be. They were delighted to find several things they could use in the Bed and Breakfast, and Stephanie felt that having a lot of Rose's things around would help make the place a success somehow. Susan knew it would help Stephanie more than it would help the place, but she just smiled at her when she said it.

A few weeks later, as the days were growing shorter Susan stood looking over the bluff that wasn't far from the building site. She could tell that the nice weather was going quick as she watched the dark clouds roll in and felt the chill in the air. "Suck it up girl," she said as she shivered a bit, remembering that long ago night yet again.

As her hand went into the pocket of her coat to pull it tighter around her, the same coat that went with the snow suit she had bought long ago and never used until now, she felt the little velvet box that she had tucked away in there and had forgotten about.

As she pulled it out all of the memories of that Christmas morning long ago with her and Tiffany together came rushing back. As she opened the box she knew what she had to do to let all the old memories dealing with Tiffany go. She took the ring out of the box and kissed it and then she flung it as hard as she could over the bluff. As she watched it go she said her good byes to Tiffany. She tucked the velvet box back into her pocket, feeling relieved and satisfied with herself; she only wished letting her other memories go was that easy.

Susan decided to head back to the site. She would tell Stephanie about throwing the ring away and letting go later, but as she came around the corner from the barn that was going up quickly and almost done she saw Stephanie talking to the foreman. Seeing Susan out of the corner of her eye, Stephanie waved her over. She forgot all about the ring as she hurried over to see if something was wrong.

"Hi honey, is something wrong?" Susan wanted to know.

"No not at all. I just wanted you to know that George tells me that he will be closing up shop and trucking all his stuff out of here by this weekend if the weather holds up long enough for him to get all his big trucks off this mountain," Stephanie said with a doubt in her eyes as she looked at the sky.

"So what does that mean?" Susan wanted to know.

"It means," Stephanie said with a huge smile on her face, "that come this weekend he's all done. It's all ours then honey, then all the real hard work will began," she said smiling at the foreman. "We can start decorating and getting it ready."

"And not a moment too soon by the looks of this sky," George interrupted, as he heard the rumble of the thunder in the distance. "They're calling for bad weather any time soon. I think we may have a solid good month or so at best of so, so weather before we are snowed under for months."

"I guess we're lucky then that the city inspectors have already given the o.k. For the heat as well as the electric," Stephanie said to him.

"True that," he said, "or else you might have waited until next spring, before they could have gotten out here. You might also want to think about getting everything you need to decorate and finish the place up, trucked up here to you before it hits. There is nothing like running out of paint with only one wall to go and no way to get more for a long time," she said with a smile.

"Great idea and you bet we will do it right away. Thanks,

I think you and your crew have done a wonderful job here," Stephanie told him. "I thank you all for the long, extra hours you put in helping us get this place livable before bad weather hit," then she gave him a wink when she said there will be big bonuses in it for everyone, he just smiled.

"I relished something this morning," Susan said as they were walking to the Jeep to head home, "I only have four more days before the deadline is up."

"What deadline?" Stephanie wanted to know.

"Remember," Susan answered, "All the papers I signed in Roberts office that day?" Seeing the perplexed look on Steph's face Susan went on. "The ones I signed with me having half ownership of all this."

"Oh, I remember," Stephanie, said, "I guess it just went out of my head with all that has been going on at the site and since I figured this is what you wanted. It is isn't it? You're not having second thoughts are you?" Stephanie asked.

"No honey, no second thoughts at all. I just remembered it this morning; I am not sure why it even came to mind. Anyway you're right, we have been so busy the last three months I have not had time to remember much either," she added with a laugh

They stayed pretty busy with the decorating and furnishing of all the rooms over the next several weeks; they had both agreed on antiques for as much of the furnishing as they could arrange so that was one less thing to decide on.

Miss Rose had a lot of great things to use, and even though Susan felt a little uneasy with the thought of it belonging to someone they knew, she didn't say anything because Stephanie seemed to think it helped her feel closer to Miss Rose.

They had decided to do themes for the rooms, a different theme or era for each room in the house, even a different color. Stephanie wasn't wild on the color idea at first, and she was afraid that would be their first real fight about the Inn, but Susan knew it would grow on Stephanie and she assured her of this.

Late while they were both relaxing on the new hearth in the sitting room, Susan was humming a tune that had plagued her all day; nothing she did made it go away.

"That is so pretty," Stephanie, said, "what song is it?"

"To tell you the truth I have no idea. I woke up with it on my mind this morning and it will not go away, and I have tried everything to get it to," Susan added.

After a few more minutes of Susan's humming, out of the blue Stephanie said, "I must say that I didn't think I could ever get use to all these new colors especially these orange walls in this room. I am more just the white wall person, but you do have pretty good taste after all darling I must say."

"It is so amazing," Susan said, looking around her, "we have gotten so much done and yet it seems like there is still so much more yet to do. Some days, I feel like we take two steps forward just to end up behind again. I think that first thing next week we should go ahead and make the trip to Kentucky that we were talking about. Just so it is done and out of the way before the winter snow blows in."

"I agree honey," Stephanie said. "I want to get the horses picked out and bought so we can have them driven out before the really bad weather hits, and I want them to get accustomed to their new home before spring."

"Did you know that I have never even been on a horse; I don't even think I have ever even been close enough to one to touch."

"Never?" Stephanie asked. "Not even when you were little."

"Nope, not once. I saw the ladies at the circus riding them once when I was small, and the church took us but

337

they seemed so huge and scary, that I just never did even want to ride one."

"Well my dear you are in for a real treat."

"Or a sore butt," Susan chimed in.

Laughing Stephanie agreed, "Yep or maybe that too, but I think you will love them nevertheless."

"I have a surprise for you," Stephanie said.

"Oh no, not another surprise, I am going to like this one right? It won't be like the surprise you gave me last month when you bought me all the material for me to build the birdhouses," she added rolling her eyes laughing.

Stephanie was holding her side from laughing so hard, "just hold on I'll be back."

She came into the room holding a yellow manila envelope out to Susan. "Here," she said, "Happy Birthday Honey."

"Hey now, how did you know it was my birthday?" she joked taking the envelope.

"A little birdie told me," Stephanie joked. "He had to tell me because he was going to freeze to death, as he is homeless, you have not built him a home yet."

"You are a jerk at times," Susan said pretending she was offended. "I would not even open this if I weren't so curious," she said as she was trying not to burst out laughing.

"Just open it," Stephanie said, "before I do."

As she ripped the flap open her hands shook as she pulled the paper out, as she read it her eyes got wide. "Oh honey, I can't believe you did this. This is the most wonderful gift anyone has ever given me," she said dropping the deed and hugging Stephanie tightly.

"I knew you loved it as much as I did when we were there so I made some phone calls right after we got home and they were in the market to sell it. I made them an offer and they signed on the dotted line. The cabin and all 198 acres are all yours baby. The hardest part was not telling you all this time. I wanted it to be a surprise but keeping it until Nov 13th was hard I am so proud of me," she said, furrowing her eyes to show Susan it was really hard. "Happy birthday darling. I hope you like it. Oh and just so you know if you don't like it, I'm keeping it myself."

"Like it!" Susan screamed, "I love it!" she said kissing Stephanie all over the face. "I felt so good being there with you, it was like the world didn't exist when we were there, I never dreamed about it being ours. I was hoping we could go back one day but I never thought that when we did it would be ours. Thank you, so much baby you are wonderful, this can now be our get away place."

"I was so hoping you would like it, but I have one more surprise for you also," Stephanie said reaching behind her back and pulling out the red file-a-folder and handing it to her.

Susan's eyes lit up as she opened the cover and read the first page and as she read what Stephanie had put in there as a dedication to her, tears were streaming down her face. "I am so glad you have finished it baby. I knew you were working on a new book but I was afraid I was taking all your time up and that you would not finish it. I feel so touched that you even dedicated it to me. My heart is so full of love and admiration for you baby."

"You're my heart Susan. Of course I would dedicate it to you, and I finished it little by little when you were over at the site or asleep. It is a love story of sorts it's all about you and I and how we met and our life from now on out. I think you will like it."

"I know I will love it," Susan said more touched than Stephanie would ever know. "I can't wait to see how it ends," she added with a smile and a kiss on Stephanie's cheek.

# CHAPTER 45

They were not in Kentucky for more than thirty minutes, when Susan fell in love with a little black colt that came running up to her while they were looking all the horses over.

Laughing the rancher said, "She wants you to rub her head. She loves it when someone scratches behind her ears." The colt nuzzled and bucked at Susan's hand trying to get her attention.

Susan looked a bit scared as she extended her hand to pet the colt, as she did her face lit up. "I have got to have this little gal Stephanie. I've just got to," she said in a baby voice.

Laughing Stephanie turned to the owner to explain this was Susan's first time ever touching a horse and to ask him about maybe buying the colt also. Before she could get it out or say anything he stopped her with a smiled and said that he would throw the colt in for free just for Susan. She seemed to love it all ready and since they were buying so many others that was the least he could do.

"I feel like a kid in a candy store here," Stephanie said, looking over and picking many of the horses she saw. "I just love horses; my Aunt Betty ran many horses over the years and I would go there as often as I could as a child."

"I have no idea what we are supposed to be looking for," Susan admitted. "I would not know a good riding horse from a bad one."

After that Susan just smiled listening to Stephanie talk to the horse rancher about growing up and being around horses when she could. She liked to hear about Steph's childhood. It was a nice childhood, one she never knew. She felt that through Steph's memory she never had to relive her own, or so she hoped.

They decided when the horse buying was done to have a nice long drive back to the airport as they had a few hours to kill before the plane was leaving, and it was such a nice bright day. The rancher had offered them lunch but they thanked him and declined.

They were driving through the green hills of a bunch of small towns when Stephanie noticed Susan became a bit quiet and sad.

"What is it?" Stephanie wanted to know. "Is something wrong honey?"

"Nothing really," Susan said, "it is just sort of a sad time for me. As we pass all these small little towns I see all these little children and it breaks my heart to pieces. Most of them are dirty and they look hungry and it just makes me sad a little, I wish I could help them."

Almost afraid to ask, Stephanie made the plunge, "Do you think it has to do with your surgery and not being able to have kids?" she asked. Trying to remain positive for

Susan they had not talked about any of it again after Susan got out of the hospital. Stephanie had tried a couple times but Susan made it clear she didn't want to talk about it. "You know I love you," she said with as much joy to her voice as she could muster, not knowing how to act when Susan got down about it or talked like that.

Looking at Steph a minute with contempt in her eyes and not knowing why it was even there, Susan said a bit loud and with a twinge of anger, "No that isn't it, it is just that they live in these little shacks and they're dirty and nasty with torn clothing that doesn't even fit, it just breaks my heart is all."

"I have been so busy looking at the trees and hills that I never even noticed the people," Stephanie began and then decided to leave it at that seeing Susan looking at her.

They drove along in silence for quite a while. They had since left Frenchburg, the last little town they went through some time back and seeing no more people or even cars on the road they each became lost in their own thoughts.

"STOP!" Susan suddenly yelled out, it was about the same time that the tiny little boy sitting on the side of the road caught Steph's attention also. As she pulled over Susan jumped out of the car before it had even stopped all the way.

Susan had so much compassion for anything and everything and it made Stephanie proud to watch her, but she didn't understand it most of the time because she didn't feel it herself that much. Oh some of Susan's compassion had rubbed off on her but not a lot. She remembered back to the day at the restaurant when Susan said she had not given having kids much thought. Seeing her now as gentle as she was with this little boy, she knew that she would have been a great mom. "Still can be," she reminded herself, "all they would need to do would be adopt."

"Hi little one," Susan said softly, as she slowly knelt down next to him so she wouldn't frighten him too much, "are you ok? Why are you sitting here on the side of the road alone like this? Are you lost?"

The little boy just stared up at her with huge scared black eyes; he didn't try to run away or even pull away and this worried Susan.

As Stephanie watched them she saw Susan stand up look around, and then, she waved her over.

"Honey come here," she called out all most in tears, "I think someone has left him out here like an animal or something."

"What did he say?" Stephanie asked hurrying over to them.

"Honey he is too little to say much. I don't know if he can even talk he has not made a sound and he is scared I can tell. He hasn't even moved he just watches. He didn't say anything not even a cry or whimper at all."

"Maybe he just wondered away from home or something," Stephanie offered hopefully. Looking around she said, "I bet he's just gotten lost or something is all."

"Look for yourself," Susan said, "there are nothing but hills and trees and wild animals around here, we have not passed a house in a long time, and the town was way back. He is no more than a baby, and I don't think a baby would or even could just wonder off like that. We have not seen a soul out here for miles not even a vehicle. If he did wonder off, then we need to help him find them; we have got to do something for him. We cannot just leave him out here."

"I know we can't just leave him here and we won't, I am just not sure what to do," Stephanie said as Susan turned to go back to the car.

"Where are you going?" Stephanie demanded. "I am going to need your help here."

"I'll be right back," Susan said over her shoulder as she went to the car, she knew she had some crackers in her back pack and she wanted to see if he was hungry. Maybe she could figure out or at least get an idea of how long he had been gone.

His eyes got even bigger when Susan offered him the crackers. "Oh honey he is starving," Susan said as she watched him devour them, "maybe that is why he isn't getting up. He looks old enough to walk at least, maybe he is just to weak to walk."

All of a sudden Susan stood up and called out, "Hello, hello, is anyone around? Can anyone hear me? I found a little boy, hello." She would wait a minute and listen before yelling again.

"Something isn't right here," Stephanie said. "I just refuse to believe that someone would just drop a child off on the side of the road. He has got to have wondered off and gotten lost; we will just find out what we need to do. We can go back to the little town we went through and ask someone what we should do."

"Well, I am not leaving him here while you figure it out. We are taking him with us. We will just miss our flight if we need to, and we can take him to town with us, cause we have got to talk to the police. I am just so mad. This poor thing, even if he is lost that is neglect," Susan said, smoothing the boy's hair a bit. "How could anyone let such a sweet thing like you go off alone?" she was saying more to herself than to the little boy.

Stephanie watched as Susan gathered the little boy into her arms and just cuddled him close to her chest. "Yes she does have a way with people," Steph thought to herself.

"It's ok sweetie," Susan said as she pulled a sweatshirt out of the bag on the back seat to put over his. "This should keep you warm," she told him. "Don't you worry we will find out what happened to you, and we will get you some food to eat first thing."

"I have some more crackers and some juice here," Stephanie said pointing to the little compartment between the seats, "try and see if he wants some more to eat, that will help hold him until we get to town and get him more to eat."

When she offered him another cracker and some juice he gobbled them down also. Stephanie noticed the tears in Susan's eyes as she just held him tight and gently rocked him while talking to him softly. She could tell that he was not as scared as he was at first, and he even started to drift off to sleep.

The ride to town was a long one. The sheriff's department was hard to find, the teenager at the gas station gave them directions and it turned out to be in the back of a little house restaurant.

Susan would not let her go there until they stopped at the one little fast food restaurant they saw on the way in. She was bound and determined to feed this boy first and she was also going to feed him as much as he could eat.

# CHAPTER 46

"Oh my," Stephanie remarked to herself as she got out of the car and looked around once they finally found the station. She bent down when she got out to talk to Susan through the car window. "Just wait in the car with him honey," looking towards the boy watching him gobble the food down for a minute, "we don't even know if anyone is here or if they can even help us. The girl that gave me directions said this Sheriff Randy was the only one that works here, but by the looks of this place he hasn't been here in a long while either."

Stephanie made her way through the over grown path to the back door and knocked, hearing nothing she knocked again. She then heard a man inside, "Come on in, don't stand out there and knock all day or you will give me a damn headache." Hearing that Stephanie went in.

"Well hello, sorry I was catching a little nap," he said a little embarrassed. "I see you're not from these parts so how can I help you young lady?" The old crusty, dingy, large, gray haired man with a beard half way down to his chest, sitting behind the little desk with his feet propped up, asked her after a rude long belch.

Stephanie noticed that he didn't have any manners and that he didn't even bother to remove his feet to the ground either.

"I hope you can help," Stephanie said, "my girlfriend and I were driving over on one of your little mountain roads, or at least, I hope it was one of yours. The best we can tell this is the closest town to where we were at when we found this little boy by the side of the road. He was just sitting there. Of course we could not just leave him there, so we have brought him here with us."

Looking around Stephanie to see if he saw anyone else and a child he said, "Well where are they?"

"They're out in the car, it's chilly and the boy had nothing on when we found him. Susan, my girlfriend, put one of her shirts over him and he was hungry, so she is feeding him right now. I didn't know if you were even in or not so I just had them wait in the car."

After having Stephanie pinpoint on the little map hanging on the wall where it was that they had found the boy, he said that he bet he was one from up at Ms Mazes place. He explained that she was a sick, bed-ridden woman that had nine kids and could never keep anyone of them at home. "I am sure the little one just got away from some of the bigger ones that was suppose to be watching him is all."

"How terrible of a mother not to know where her kids are, and in this weather no less," Stephanie said, more under her breath than to him.

He heard her anyway and said, "Sweetheart, that's a common occurrence around here, a fact of life here in the boonies," he added with a wink.

She stood there in disbelief with her mouth open as he just calmly wrote some information on a piece of paper and handed it to her.

"What is this?" Stephanie asked as she read the little paper that he had handed her.

"This is Ms. Maze's address and directions to her little place. She doesn't have a phone so I can't call her, just take the child there and see if he is hers."

Shocked that he was saying what she was hearing him say to her, "How do you even know he belongs there? Are you not even going to come and look at him to see if you know him? What the hell are we to do with him, if the little boy doesn't belong to her?" she asked.

"Then bring him back here and we will go from there if he doesn't belong there. I would not know if he did or not just by looking at the kid anyway, they all look alike to me. I am sure he is hers as she is the only one that lives within twenty miles of where you found him, and I don't see no little thing like that going further than that."

She was still stunned and shaking her head as she walked to the car, not believing what all he had said to her and how he had handled the whole thing, as she got into the car Susan could tell something was wrong.

"I cannot believe that son of a bitch," Stephanie said as she handed the paper to Susan for her to read, "I have not been so mad in a long time, can you believe it? I could bite through nails right about now."

Looking at the paper dumbfounded Susan said nothing, she just let Stephanie rant on. This was the maddest Susan had ever seen her.

"That poor kid, we now have to run and try to see if this is even his mom and if it is then why? So he can get away again when it is freezing cold and then die, I don't mind taking him there it isn't that, don't get me wrong. I just cannot believe this Sheriff, how does he know we are good people and will not just run off with him. How does he know anything?" she said, almost in tears.

"Honey, I am sure he trusts us to at least do what ever he wants us to do. After all, we did bring the baby to the station in the first place; if we were bad people would we have showed our face and taken him to the police in the first place? Now slow down and tell me what all he said," Susan coaxed.

"I know you're right baby," Stephanie said as she looked at the little boy in her lovers arms, "I just cannot believe the sheriffs uncaring attitude towards all this, I mean for heavens sakes he's just a little child," she said, rubbing his back.

Susan was stunned and in tears when Stephanie told her what the sheriff had said to her and what he said for them to do.

"How in the world can his mother be like this, sick or not I don't care, it isn't right. She should have someone come in to help her out, some family or friends or someone. This just breaks my heart."

The rest of the ride was mostly in silence. "You know what?" Susan said as they pulled into the little dirt road drive. It was marked by huge potholes, which seemed to wind forever. Before leading up to the little shack. "Have you noticed he never makes a sound, he doesn't cry or whimper or anything."

Stephanie had noticed but didn't want to say anything, she had not been around many kids in her life, but the ones she had been around she remembered cried all the time and was very loud. She was afraid if she voiced that concern or let on like she was worried that it would upset Susan even more. So she said, "Maybe he is just too scared," she offered, "or even in shock, you know it had to be traumatic for such a little thing."

"Maybe," Susan said not believing it for a minute. As they pull up and stopped in front of the little run down shack that was not fit for one person let alone a large family, Susan could barely see someone inside. There was no light on though, and it was so quiet even eerily quiet that she didn't know what to do next. "What should we do?" she said to Stephanie.

"Let's go in," Stephanie said given her hand a little squeeze. "We came all this way, and we need to see if he even belongs here. If not we will need time to get him back to town before it gets too dark and everything closes up around here. I have a feeling things don't stay open very late, and I can bet the sheriff doesn't stay there a minute longer then he needs to." she said trying to smile.

"Ok," Susan said, "lets go, but I am keeping that shirt on him." He was asleep so she tried to not jostle him too much so he would not wake up.

# CHAPTER 47

Susan was hugging the boy tightly to her chest trying to not wake him, darkness was setting in and it seemed even darker up this holler with no streetlights around. Boards were sticking up all over the porch and it was all Stephanie could do to catch herself as she stumbled when her foot got stuck under one of them.

As Susan was about to knock on the flimsy torn up screen door a little girl swung open the door, "ello," she said with a twang so thick in her accent that made it hard to tell what she was saying. She also had the same big black eyes as the little boy that was in her arms still fast asleep Susan noticed.

"Hi honey. Is your mommy here?" Susan asked. "We need to talk to her if we could please."

"Ya' she's back thar in the bed," she said pointing into the house. "Come in let me show you whar she's at."

They both thought it odd that the little girl made no mention at of the little boy that Susan was still holding tight.

They both heard a voice call out from the back of the little shack, "Heather, who it is out thar?"

"It's some ladies mama, thar not from these parts causin' I don't know them frum round here. I'm bringin' um back."

The little girl pulled open some curtains so they could go through, "she's right thar," the little girl said, pointing in the dark room, "go'on in."

"Heather git'em some drink child, mine yore manners."

"No thank you," they both said at the same time.

"We just came to talk to you about this little boy we found along side of a road earlier. It was about seven miles from here, we were just in town and the sheriff said we should see you to find out if he lives here or not," Stephanie said

"What ya got thar?" the lady asked.

"Are you Maze?"

"Yes'um I am, is that little Billy you got thar? Have you a seat right thar."

Susan about tripped over something on the floor and said.

"It's hard to see anything," she remarked, "would it be ok if we turned on a light?"

"Ain't got no lights out here, no electricity ya know? Heather fetch us the lantern in here want ya?"

"Yes'um, I'll bring it right away mama," she said as she hurried out of the room to get the lantern. They watched as she brought it back in and sat it on the little table next to the bed before running out again.

"So you fount little Billy did ya? One of the youngins tells me last night he went a wonderin' off again. He's mute every since he came down real sick, so when he goes a wonderin' like that you got to just trip over him or you cant hardly find him. That's why itsa so quiet in here, some of'em are off a lookin' for him now. I reckon they ain't going to find him now though."

Both women were in shock to hear this woman talk, not from her accent or from how ignorant she sounded but from the lack of caring in her words and voice for this little boy that wonders off a lot to hear her tell it.

"Begging your pardon ma'am," Stephanie cut in. "I do not mean to judge you or judge how you raise your children but it seems to me, that you should make sure he isn't out of your sight so he can not just wonder off like that, especially with him being handicapped and so young. If you have not noticed it is getting pretty cold outside most days. It is the middle of November after all, it may seem like Indian summer around here during the day but I know it gets cold at night. When we found him he didn't have anything on, not a diaper or shirt or anything, and he was cold and starving. He ate everything we gave him like he had not eaten in days. You said they told you he has been gone since last night. So you mean to say he had been gone all night long. A little thing like that had to spend the night alone outside. It's a wonder he didn't freeze to death. I bet no one even thought about calling the sheriff in to look for him either did they?" She was angry now and raising her voice.

"Listen here lil' missy," the woman interrupted, "I ain't had no schoolin' to speak of and I'm a sick woman, I can't be runnin' after this little bastard ever time he wonders off. Don't ya'll come in my house and lay judgment cross me when you don't know nothin' bout nothin' that goes on round here."

"Well excuse me but I do know enough to know not to have more babies when I can't even feed the ones I got. I know enough to know not to have more babies when I am too sick to take care of them properly, and I would know enough to watch any babies I had if I had any of my own that is," Stephanie said, even more angry. "Hell if you need to tie him to you or one of the big kids so he can't wonder off, how hard would that be? He is your son for goodness sakes woman, take care of him."

"Lil' Billy isn't my baby anywaze, he's my grand baby. His mama is my 12-year-old daughter, she was raped by some ugly ole man up the road a piece and now we's got lil' Billy. We gotta make do with what we got he's just another mouth to feed anywaze. Thank ya for bringin' him here now get back in yore vehicle and move on out fore I have Timmy take after you with the shot gun."

Stephanie hurriedly got to her feet to leave the room, reaching for the baby from Susan she startled him when she took him out of her arms waking him up she then put him on the floor as she grabbed Susan's hand, "come on, we are getting out of this fucked up place."

357

Susan would not budge when Stephanie pulled at her, "Please go on out to the car," Susan said, "I will be out in a minute, I want to talk to her for a minute."

"Hell no, I am not leaving this room without you with me. Now come on, this woman is nuts and that's about the nicest thing I can think to say about her right now. The boy lives here even if he doesn't belong here so lets go, we did what we could."

"No," Susan said. "Please go outside. I will be there in a minute. Please baby for me."

Stunned Stephanie just looked at her and then without saying a another word marched out of the room; they heard her slam the front door as well as the car door.

Susan was stunned and silent for a minute, more in shock at all that had been said by both women then anything else. This wasn't how she envisioned this meeting to go at all.

"Ms Maze," she said as she found her voice again, "I am sorry and I am sure Stephanie didn't mean what she said, and I know she didn't mean to judge you, she isn't that sort of person. I know she did not mean half of what she was saying. We are just worried about the baby, and I know that is no excuse to come in here to your house and act like that so I will not make excuses for her, but I would like to apologize for her behavior."

She could tell the woman was listening to what she was saying so she went on. "We are not from around here as you know, and we are just use to different things and a different way of life is all. Billy is such a sweet baby and I mean it when I say if you ever need anything, anything at all you call me." Looking through her backpack she pulled out her business card and handed it to her, "This is my home number and address, please call for any reason. You can call me collect any time you would like," she added. She could see there was a tear in the woman eyes. "Are you ok?" Susan asked.

The woman spent a lot of time telling her all about her illness and about all the kids and about her man dying in the coalmines a couple years ago leaving them with nothing at all except the little shack they were in, and she also told Susan about her illness and about how she was too ill and not able to work at all.

Susan's heart was breaking as the woman talked and told her the whole story. She also kept hearing Stephanie blow the horn several times but ignored her.

When the woman just sat there after she finished her story in silence Susan rummaged in her purse again and pulled out all the money she had with her.

"Here," she said handing the woman a wad of money, wishing it could be a lot more.

"No ma'am I can't take yore money," she said.

"Please ma'am, take it, at least take it for the kids sake," Susan said, "and please remember, I do mean if you need anything at all I would like to help. Please forgive my girlfriend; she isn't a mean person at all. If you don't mind I am going to write down your address before I go."

"No, I'on't mind," the woman, said with tears in her eyes again. "Yore an angel and I wont ever forgets you or yore kine spirit."

Susan leaned over and gave her a long tender hug, "take care of yourself," she whispered.

The lady watched and was touched by her caring as she bent down to little Billy and picked him up.

"Hey little fellow, I am so glad I got to meet you. You're a special little man, and I sure am going to miss you." She said as she gave him a big tight hug, "now don't go wondering off anymore, you have got to stay home to help grandma out around here when you grow up and get bigger," she said with a smile as she kissed his nose. "And the next time I am around here I am going to come see you, so be a good boy," she said with tears streaming down her face as she hugged him tight again.

Putting him down she turned back to the woman and said,

"He didn't have anything on when we found him and his skin was ice cold, so I gave him my favorite sweater that I had with me. Do you think it will be ok for him to keep it and maybe sleep in so I know he is warm at night?"

"Shore is," she said, "shore its ok."

Susan felt a little bit better about things as she went through the quiet dark house back outside onto the porch just as Stephanie blew the horn again.

As Susan got in the car she could see Stephanie was ready to pounce with questions. Holding up her hand she said, "Before you say a word Stephanie I don't want to talk about it at all right now, ok?"

"Fine," was all Stephanie said dying to know what had happened or been said; now wishing she had waited in the house with her.

Susan was sitting with her arms crossed feeling very empty without little Billy in them now just watching the night roll in over the hills as they drove out of the long dark holler. She saw some children's figures come over a hill into a clearing on the other side of the hills, and as she watched she wondered which one of the children was little Billy's mother.

All the way to the airport Susan could not get her mind off the family she had just met. She knew she had to do something to help them out but she wasn't sure what yet, and she didn't know if Stephanie would even be willing to help. She decided to keep it to herself, at least for now.

They had missed their plane by the time they got to the airport, but was lucky enough to get the next one out that same night. Stephanie was relieved that they didn't need to wait until the morning as she had enough of this place for one trip. She didn't think her emotions could take anymore, she was glad to be getting back home. She could tell Susan was still thinking about the little boy, and she wanted to help get her mind off of him. It was over and there was nothing they could do now, and she hoped getting back home and finishing up the ranch would help.

"You will have your hands full learning how to train your new baby colt," Stephanie said to try and pull Susan's mind out of where it was.

"I know and I am so excited about it. I want to learn all I can about horses in general; I think we need to hire a good stable hand that knows a lot about horses; they can help me with them and show me how to train them also."

Stephanie was happy that Susan now seemed to have her mind on something else and no longer just on the trip. The flight was a bit bumpy, and she was not feeling well with flying right now. As they hit an air bump or turbulence as the pilot called it, Stephanie grabbed Susan's hand.

"I don't care what he calls it, I call it just get me on the ground soon," Stephanie said through her teeth that she was grinding together now giving Susan cold chills, she hated that sound.

Susan had been so lost in her thoughts she had forgot that Stephanie didn't like to fly, and as she grabbed her hand she realized how bumpy it really was. "I am so sorry honey. I know you don't like to fly; it won't be long now we are just outside of Colorado. If you want to try and sleep it might make you feel better," she offered.

"Hell no, I do not want to sleep. I want to get there so we can land, when my feet are on the ground I will feel better and not until then. Just let me squeeze your hand and I will be fine," she said without so much as a smile.

As they touched down the plane did a little hopping before coming to rest. It was one of the worse landings Susan had ever been on and Susan saw tears in Stephanie eyes. Susan knew she pretended to be strong about everything but this was one thing she knew scared her to death, and Susan made a mental note to try to drive more and less flying for Stephanie's sake.

# CHAPTER 48

Their trip to Kentucky as well as the family they had met there stayed heavily on Susan's mind for several days after they returned home; she knew she had to do something.

When she figured out what she wanted to do she never let Stephanie know. She was not sure how she would react if she knew that she had gotten a huge care box together loaded with everything from clothing to food to money, and she knew she would not have found out had it not been for Lilly at the post office.

When she struggled to carry the huge box into the post office one morning Lilly rushed to help her carry it and she could not help herself, she had to ask about it.

"So tell me dear, what do we have here?"

Susan not wanting to tell her felt she had no other choice but to tell her what she was doing and why.

After Susan told Lilly about finding the little boy and the family they had met there and how the whole town was like that and needed help.

Lilly thought Susan had such a great idea with her wanting to help the family out that lived so far away and all that Lilly said she wanted to do it on a bigger scale and make it all year around not just for the holiday season. She decided that she would start spreading the word around town, to see how many people would be willing to help out with adopting this family.

By the time Lilly was done. The entire town knew and most everyone had it planned out as to who would be sending what box on what day and she had it on going to help this family out for as long as they needed help.

"I have a great idea," Susan said as she was talking to Lilly one day about their project a couple weeks after they had started sending stuff to the family, "why don't we see if we can't get a list of all the families in that town that need our help. We can help so many more families, and we have so many people in this town willing to help us out. We can get all the information such as how many kids there are per families and their sizes etc. we can then give each person here that wants to sort of adopt a family of there on all the information they will need to be able to help them out, what do you think?"

Lilly loved the idea. She said she liked how it people from here adopting a whole family there, and she said she was going to name it K.A.W.S. for "Keeping America Warm and Safe, one family at a time" and that it would be Susan's project.

"You're such a special woman," Lilly said out of the blue while they were making plans, "I know Miss Rose would have loved you and love that you and Stephanie found one another. She had a lot of love and compassion in her heart for others just like you, most people don't even know that about her because she did go around others much but I knew her and I saw it. You just don't see that now days."

Susan was at a loss for words and she was very touched and felt excepted by this woman, "Thank you," Susan whispered before going on, "ok," she said. "Getting back to what we need to do first. We have decided to get in touch with the Sheriff and get a list of all the families in town that could use a helping hand from time to time, right?" Lilly shook her head yes so Susan made the phone call.

He was more than happy to fax them the names and addresses as well as all the information he could get on each family. He wasted no time either, they had all the information they needed the next day. He had, like everyone else had, already heard what a wonderful thing the tiny town in Colorado was doing for the one family all ready, and what they wanted to do for all who needed it in that tiny town in Kentucky. He spent all day and night tracking down all the information he could and getting all the families signed up that wanted or needed loving help.

It also came to Susan's attention that one of the older ladies in town had a niece that lived about thirty-five miles away from the little town in Kentucky, and that she thought it was a great idea what they were doing in helping out. She herself wanted to help out in any way she could, so she agreed to go on the weekend to help them out. She was studying to be a nurse and with only six more months to go before she was an LPN, she felt this would help her career as well as help the family's out. She would give them all free check ups, she also said her boyfriend was a carpenter and he was willing to go with her on the weekends and help them fix the places up, even add some rooms here and there with no charge.

Susan had let Lilly know that she would pay for anything that the families needed that the other people could not afford or that wasn't covered when they were helping out. All she had to do was let her know, and she wanted to buy all the building materials also.

She was very worried as to how Stephanie would take the news when she heard about it. It had grown out of her control, and it was on such a huge scale now she was surprised Stephanie had not heard about it yet. She knew she had to tell her because there was going to be a big write-up in the paper next week, and she didn't want her to find out that way; she just didn't know when she would.

It was late in the evening about three weeks after they had first started sending things to the families in Kentucky when Stephanie came up to her as she was doing the dishes after dinner and just hugged her.

"Wow I like that, what was it for?" Susan asked.

"I just think you're wonderful baby. You have done such a wonderful thing for that family and even that whole town now. I would never have even thought of it myself. You have started something that has all ready and will continue to change so many lives there and here as well. Some of these older people didn't have a lot to live for anymore around here, and now you have given them whole family to live for and help. You said you wished you could do something to help and now look at it I am so impressed with you."

Susan felt so much pride in herself as she heard Stephanie talk. "I knew I had to figure out a way to help not only that family but also as many others as I could. It wasn't all me, honey the whole town did most of it."

Susan didn't realize how proud of her Stephanie was as she stood back and watched her finish the dishes up. She had thought that when the horses were delivered a few days after they got home from Kentucky that Susan's mind would have been on them instead of on the family they had met. Susan didn't say anything about it but Stephanie knew she had been thinking of them off and on when she would catch her lost in thought, but Stephanie never dreamed she would have been instrumental in making such an elaborate plan as she had came up with to help not just that family but many others also. Susan and Lilly had done a wonderful job, and Susan never missed a beat either. She learned all she could about the horses and she even started training the little black colt herself as well as helping care for all the other horses each day.

About a week later Susan received a short letter from Maze that was very hard to read. She then knew she had done the right thing, if she had ever had any doubts she no longer did.

Susan could make out only part of the letter, she knew that it was mostly a thank you to her and the whole town and that she was very touched with the kindness that they all was showing, saying that they had really made a difference in many families in her town. She was also sending her an invitation to return anytime for a visit. There was something else written in there about the baby but that was lost to Susan. She just could not make out what she had tried to write; she could not make it out at all. She felt touched that Ms. Maze had taken it upon herself to try and write the letter alone. That meant a lot to Susan, it made her feel good that she could help them out.

Christmas was now fast approaching and the house was pretty much done other than a few things here and there. They had decided to make the main living quarters on the back end of the Inn so they could have a panoramic view of the mountains. They even had glass windows from floor to ceiling added throughout most of the house at Susan's insistence as she loved to look at the snow capped mountains.

"Honey," Susan called out to Stephanie as she came out of the house, "I am going to run into town and get some Christmas decorations for us to put up I'll be back later."

"Great, get a lot of the fake snow for the windows, you know how we don't get enough of that around here," she teased Susan.

"Oh you're just so funny," Susan said, giving her a peck on the cheek, "Oh before I forget, you a had call this morning when you was out at the stables. I tried to put it through but the line was tied up out there, so I took a message and it is in by the phone," she said with a wave of her hand as she got in the new 4x4 SUV that she had bought for herself a few weeks back.

The drive to town was a peaceful one for Susan as she made plans all during the drive. She planned to spend the next few weeks planning out activities that their future guests could do while staying there. They had decided to not start taking in guests until after all the holidays were over with, as this was their first holiday together and they wanted to spend it alone and also not to feel rushed about getting everything else done. So she was in no hurry.

They had hired their stable keeper all ready, but they still needed a handy man and grounds keeper as well as someone to run their little guest shop/store and the coffee shop.

All that soon changed when Susan got back home that evening with a back end full of Christmas decorations. I think I got all the decorations they had in town," Susan said getting out of the SUV as Stephanie came running out to meet her.

"We got it," Stephanie said interrupting Susan. Waving a piece of paper in the air. "Honey, look, we got it," she repeated again excited.

"What ever are you talking about?" Susan asked, "come on and walk with me honey and you can tell me what you are talking about," she said, "I need to brush Courtney down before it gets to dark."

Stephanie walked with Susan to the stables and watched as she was brushing Courtney down, before going on with what she was saying. Courtney was her already spoiled rotten black colt, of no fault of Susan's; at least that is what she told everyone even as she snuck sugar cubes out to her.

"Honey we got our first reservation," Stephanie said, smiling from ear to ear, "I just got off the phone with them a little bit ago. There the ones that call this morning and left the message, it's a group of eighteen lesbians and they're going to stay for a month. They will be here two weeks before Christmas and stay until January 15th."

"Honey, that's next week and we're not even ready. We still have so much to finish and do first. We have got to hire some more help and we have got to plan things for them to do. We have not even named the ranch yet or anything, and now we have a ton of decorations to put up," Susan interjected with desperation creeping into her voice. "I didn't even know we were advertising for this year at all. I thought we had decided that we were going to wait until after the holidays to start taking reservations at all?"

"January was the earliest to start booking so we would have a few more weeks to get ready, and have to ourselves. When they called I could not turn them down, they read that no reservations were going to be taken until January in the flyer, but they told me that they needed a place before that and could we please make an exception? They said this group does this twice each year and if they like it here they will want to come back next summer, so how could I turn that down? So of course I said yes."

"Honey, there is just so much left for us to do," Susan interjected. She was starting to feel overwhelmed, "there is way more here to do for us two for the next three weeks; and now it is down to getting it all done in one week."

"I know there is, and I know I said not until the first of the year that is why I made sure I had all their information. If you want me to call them back and cancel I could do that, but as it is only a week away I will need to call them today so they can try and find somewhere else. They had plans that fell through when where they was going to stay burnt down so that leaves them with nowhere to go if we say no. It is only a few weeks early, we can handle it can't we honey?"

Susan shrugged her shoulders pretending to be mad, she knew Steph was pleading their case hard, so she had to give her a bit of a hard time. Seeing the look on Steph's face she started laughing, "I am only kidding," she said, "of course it's ok but we've got a whole lot to do before they get here, and we have like no time to do it. Next time be warned guilt will not work on me either," she said smiling, "you better hope Johnnie agrees to help us out also," she said as she put Courtney's brush up. "We have activities to arrange, parties to plan, supplies to buy," patting Courtney's head, she whispered to her to let her know she would be back later to finish up.

They walked to the little gazebo by the side of the huge house so they could sit and talk. Susan loved the little swing they had added to the center of it. It had quickly become her favorite spot to just get away to think or read.

"First things first," Susan said, "We have got to think of a name for this ranch. Robert called and wanted the name of this place weeks ago so he could have it added to the records at the courthouse. If we had a name we could add the name to the flyers and to all the advertising you have been doing," she added with a smile. "Do you have any ideas on one?"

Stephanie thought for a minute and then said, "I have a couple of ideas for some names, why don't we each tell a couple names that we like, and then, we can go from there. We can pick the one we like the best."

"Great idea," Susan agreed, "I have given it some thought and I was thinking of something like, "The Come

Again Ranch" or "The Fliberdjibbet Ranch" or even something like "The Flibberty Jibberty Ranch."

Laughing Stephanie asked, "How in the world did you think of names such as these? I like those names don't get me wrong, they're a little weird but I like them. I was thinking more like "Smell the Roses Ranch" or "Stop and Smell the Roses Ranch", you know, simple like that and also something in Rose's memory."

"See those are good ones also," Susan said, "So how do you want to decide this? We have picked such different names."

"I have no idea; I guess we could just write them down and draw them out of a hat or something corny like that," Stephanie said as a joke.

"That's not corny at all. I think that is a great idea," Susan said as she jumped up, "let me run and get some paper and a pen; I'll be right back."

"Don't forget the hat," Stephanie yelled to Susan's back laughing.

"All I can find honey is your cowboy hat and a ball cap so it's your pick, which one do you want to go with?" she said holding both of them out for Stephanie to pick one.

"I think the cowboy hat would be fitting," Stephanie said after thinking about it for a minute, "let's use the cowboy hat as we are christening the ranch with its own name after all. Get it? Ranch, cowboy hat," she said smiling at Susan.

"Yes I get it," Susan said laughing, "and I agree with you, I think the cowboy hat is the one we should use."

"I can't believe we are picking the name of our ranch out of a hat," Stephanie said still laughing. "I wonder if this is how they did it in the old Wild West?"

"I sort of doubt that they did it that way," Susan said," but I think it is a wonderful idea and who knows, come to think of it they just might have decided the fate of the names of the ranches this very way. You're just a genius for thinking of it," she added, kissing Stephanie on the cheek.

They both decided to use Johnnie as the official name drawer. She had been with them now as their stable keeper for only a few short weeks, but they could tell she was the right woman for the job because she was so great with the horses, and Susan felt like she was learning a lot from her.

It didn't take them long to locate her; she was on the phone in the bunkhouse talking with her nephew. So after getting her attention to let her know when she was done to come outside and see them, they needed her help to do something for them. They decided to go for a walk around the stables.

It wasn't long before Johnnie joined them in the stables.

"You wanted to see me?" Johnnie said in her Texas drawl, as that was where she was from.

"Yes, we need you to do a couple things for us and with us, first here's the plan," Stephanie said to Johnnie, "we want to name the ranch tonight as we have guests coming

375

to stay here with us in under a week. We have some names all ready picked out and wrote on little papers in the hat. We were wondering if you would be so kind as to pick us one name out of the hat. This way you have a hand in what this place is called also, right along with us. Then after that we have a lot to do to finish getting ready for the guests so we were wondering, with a nice pay raise of course, if you would be willing to help out with getting everything around here done and ready. I am sure with your help we can be ready for them in time. All eighteen of them," she added with a desperate look on her face.

Seeing the cowboy hat she had to smile, "It's befitting I think to name the ranch out of this hat," she said taking the hat out of Susan's hand, "and sure I will be happy, no I'd be honored to pick the name out for you all. I will also be more then glad to help you all get ready, and I do not need a pay raise for helping either, but now if you want to give me a huge bonus as my Christmas gift I would not mind," she added with a wink, "and I do think with us all three working we can get this place ready by next week, now first things first, how does this work? Is it the first name I pick out going to be the winner no matter what?"

Both women looked at one another and agreed, "Yes, first one you draw out will be our new name here on the ranch."

They had both wrote the names that they had picked out down on little pieces of paper that Susan tore out of the tablet all ready, and they were in the hat just waiting,

Johnnie shuffled the little pieces of paper around in the hat for a minute before saying. "Ok you guys ready?" she asked.

They both shook their heads yes, they were very excited and could hardly wait.

As she drew out a piece of paper she put the hat down and slowly opened the paper up. She burst out laughing at the name she read to herself.

"She must have picked one of yours," Stephanie said with a smile at Susan. "Ok lets hear it," she said looking at Johnnie; I know it is one of hers as she had the funny names picked out, which one will it be?

Clearing her throat Johnnie went on very dramatically. "Forever more from here on out this ranch will now be known as The Flibberty Jibberty Rose Ranch."

Smiling Stephanie said, "I love it baby but wait a minute, that isn't one of the names you had picked out all ready I would have remembered it."

"Yes it is," Susan said, "I was just very touched that you wanted Rose's name as part of the ranches name, so I added it to all mine when we wrote them down on the papers just in case one of mine got picked."

"Come here woman," Stephanie said as she pulled Susan into her arms, "I love you very much and I love the name. Thank you," she whispered into the night, "this one is for you Rose."

# CHAPTER 49

"I have an idea," Johnnie interrupted their quite moment. When she saw she had both their attention she went on, "I was just on the phone with my nephew Wayne, he was bummed out because his band was suppose to play a big gig in the Springs this weekend but now it has just been canceled because they got some local group from the Springs called Bone Farm to come in instead of them."

"That sucks," Susan said, "why would they do that to them?"

"Who knows, I guess they just thought it would draw a bigger crowd in as they're more well known, more money maybe. What I was thinking is we should throw a big shindig up here this weekend and invite the whole town. Anything we don't get done we could have helpers, and the boys group is called Fatal Sin. They could do all the music and the three of us could host the whole thing; it would be great fun," she added.

"I think that is a great idea," Susan said after Johnnie paused to take a breath. "We could christen the ranch with its new name during the party. Another thing that we could do instead of taking the time to put all the decorations up ourselves, we could make it a decorating party also and let everyone help." she added. "So what do you both think?"

I think it is a great idea and will help the town feel more a part of this place also," Stephanie offered. "But it will only give us two days to get everything ready for the party; do you two think we can do it by Saturday? And that also leaves less time to get ready for our guests that will be arriving next week."

"Sure I know we can," they both chimed in at the same time.

"A little hard work and some elbow grease and we will be ready," Johnnie offered as reassurances.

"Ok then," Stephanie went on, "I will do the flyers and pass them around, Lilly can help me get the word out."

She is really good at that Susan chimed in with a wink to Stephanie.

"I know there is a town meeting tomorrow evening and most everyone will be there so I will have Lilly announce it then," Stephanie said. "Johnnie, you will need to contact Fatal Sin and let them know, and Susan you can buy all the food we will need. Now did I leave anything out?" Stephanie asked as she frantically racked her brain to make sure no stone was left uncovered.

"Aye, Aye, Captain," they both said in unison again with a laugh.

"Dang if I knew you were such a slave driver I may have not taken this job," Johnnie said teasing her, "and I can't think of anything that you might have left out," she added.

"Or you could have just asked for more money," Susan offered, "If you knew she was so demanding."

"Now, now ladies, this is not gang up on poor little Stephanie day," she said teasing them both. "Johnnie, first I need for you to give me all the boys names, and what they do in the band so I can put them in the flyers," Stephanie said getting her notebook out.

"Lets see, Wayne is the lead singer, and helps write songs. If I am not mistaken I think he also plays the rhythm guitar some, then there is Shawn he writes as well as plays the drums, he also sings back up for Wayne and Raymond is the lead guitarist. They have been together now for a little over two years playing their own stuff as well as others. They are really good and it has been a few months since I last heard them, and I know they are just going to love this," she added.

The next two days were so busy that they flew by. Stephanie had been right about Lilly, she had been phenomenal in getting the word out to everyone. She had even taken it upon herself to have them RSVP to her so she could keep count of who all was coming and who was bringing what with them. They had decided to let it be a potluck barbeque on Lilly's suggestion, less work for them and it made people feel needed also. Susan and Stephanie were going to supply all the meats and everyone else was bringing a side dish or desserts of some kind.

Johnnies' nephew, Wayne, as well as the rest of the band were just ecstatic. She had even promised them part of any bonus she got out of this, but they refused it, saying they would love to do it just for practice, and to help them out.

Before they knew it Saturday, was here and it was just a matter of time before the people started arriving. They had done it with not a minute to spare by the time the cars and trucks and even a few tractors started rolling up the mountain road. Every thing was just perfect, the band was warming up their new equipment off to the side where Johnnie and Stephanie had made them a make shift stage out of the flat bed wagon. Stephanie even surprised them with new mikes as well as a new sound system.

Susan had the meat cooking at full blast on several of the huge grills out back, and the weather could not have been nicer for an early winters' evening.

As Susan was dishing out the hot dogs and hamburgers to all the kids, she could not believe how many people showed up. She had not seen this many people all together before in her life. She knew if they ever did this again, someone else was in charge of the grills she thought to herself with a smile.

Everyone had pitched right in with hanging the decorations up and they got it done in no time at all.

As Stephanie called for everyone's attention, Susan could not have been happier. Even when Johnnie came to help her with the food it didn't seem to help, she was exhausted in a good way but exhausted never the less.

"Hello, may I please have everyone's attention?" Stephanie called over the mike again, this time everyone quieted down and offered her their full attention. "I want everyone to welcome my woman Susan to the stage and also our wonderful stable keeper and helper Johnnie to the stage. We are going to christen this ranch with its new name this evening so if everyone will give them a big round of applause, we can get them up here and get started."

They were both embarrassed as they made their way to the home made wagon stage, with all the applauding going on around them.

When they were up on stage, thanks to the help of Wayne and Shawn the crowd quieted down, eager to hear the new name. There were several bets going around about what the name would be so they all wanted to be sure that they could hear it when it was read.

As Stephanie read the new name of the ranch there was a lot of laughter from the crowd below. As it was a funny name after all, and then as it struck some of them as to what it meant they all cheered. Not a single person told them they didn't like it so they figured that was pretty good, and many even told then that they liked it a lot, and they thought it had a nice meaning.

As it grew late, everyone started saying their good-byes to each other as well as to them and making their way to their vehicles to head back down the mountain, after all they still had church tomorrow.

"This could not have been a more perfect night," Stephanie said after the party wrapped up, taking Susan in her arms walking with her to their spot on the swing she went on saying, "the christening of the ranches new name went well and everyone is going home stuffed and happy, except for a few men that bet on the name. They're not quite as happy, but they will get over it," she added with a wink. "Can you believe one man bet we would name this the Lick A Lot Ranch?" with that they both busted out laughing, then Stephanie went on, "We did it honey, our first real party together," she added.

She and Susan sat on the swing watching the long line of taillights go back down the mountain as the party winded down.

"I think we should do this every year to celebrate the ranches birthday. We could plan it the same time each year and either not take boarders at all during that time, or just let them know what will be going on around here, so they can join if they wish too. This way the town folks will feel more like they're part of us also," Susan suggested.

"Great idea honey. I agree to let it be so," she said as a joke with a giggle, as she laid her head on Susan's shoulder, "I love loving you, I hope you know this?"

"I love that too and I love loving you also," she added with a smile and a soft kiss.

They both heard the phone ringing in the background as they sat cuddling and kissing on the swing.

"Who ever could that be?" Susan asked, "Every one from town was here or so it seemed anyway, and I don't think many have had time to get back home yet," she added.

A few minutes later Johnnie came out onto the porch and called out, "Susan, telephone for you, it's some frantic woman, she's hysterical and very hard to understand. There isn't a good connection on the other end of the line. She said it's an emergency, come quick."

Looking at Steph for a second, with a worried look on her face Susan jumped up and ran to the phone.

*The End*

*Now Just*

*Hold on, not so fast*

*There's more to come.*

*"In the next book."*

*Byeeee.*

# About the Author

Raised on a farm in Kentucky Ms. Chatelain has worked and volunteered for many years as a crisis intervention counselor. She is an excellent Mum to her two teenagers as well as an author and accomplished artist. Several of her paintings have been shown in galleries. She focuses her works on the female body through her art as well as her words. Her spare time is spent helping the homeless through a mission she started with her family. She touches everyone she meets in one-way or the other. Ms. Chatelain lives in North Carolina with her family. *Around We Go* is her first novel; she is currently working on the second novel in this series, *Around We Go Again.*

Printed in the United States
1078700001B/20

9 781403 313775